CW00708005

BEHAVIOUR THERAPY NURSING

Behaviour Therapy Nursing

PHILIP J. BARKER
Clinical Nurse Specialist: Behaviour Therapy,
Tayside Area Clinical Psychology Department,
Royal Dundee Liff Hospital,
Dundee, Scotland

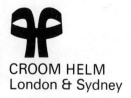

CROOM HELM
London & Sydney

© 1982 Philip Joseph Barker
Reprinted 1985

Croom Helm Ltd, Provident House, Burrell Row,
Beckenham, Kent BR3 1AT

Croom Helm Australia Pty Ltd, Suite 4, 6th Floor,
64-76 Kippax Street, Surry Hills, NSW 2010, Australia

British Library Cataloguing in Publication Data

Barker, Philip J.
    Behaviour therapy nursing.
    1. Behaviour therapy
    I. Title
    616.89'142   RC489.B4

    ISBN 0-7099-0637-4

Typeset by Leaper & Gard Ltd, Bristol
Printed and bound in Great Britain by
Biddles Ltd, Guildford and King's Lynn

CONTENTS

FOREWORD

The author's work has been known to me for some years. I have heard him speak, read his articles and examined his students, so the high quality of this text has not come as a surprise. Even so, I was not prepared for the scope of the work and the depth and breadth of the subject.

Readers should perhaps start with the last chapter, which could more appropriately be called a *credo* than an epilogue. In this chapter the author outlines his theoretical stance, draws a map of the territory which is explored and reveals his humanistic attitude and his moral principles. He is convinced that the therapist's relationship with the patient plays a large part in influencing the outcome of treatment and throughout the book he demonstrates that the therapist mirrors, in his work, the relationship he, in his student days, had developed with his mentor.

The subject matter of the book is immensely broad, spanning, as it does, the social psychology of learning, or behaviourism, of inter-action and motivation. The quotations which head each chapter introduce the author to his readers as a veritable Renaissance man.

The author makes the subject appear beautifully simple, almost like common sense. The reader is treated with great respect and credited with the desire and the ability to create an integrated whole from the detailed information he is offered. The title of the book does perhaps not really do justice to the text, which has much wider application than is usually associated with the term 'behaviour modification'. An analogy is drawn with the nursing process, but it would be more accurate to say that what has been spelled out is what the nursing process is really all about. Explanation of what is involved in assessment alone occupies nearly one-third of the book and it makes one realise how glibly some nurses embark on a care plan after only a most cursory assessment. Three people with very different problems are used as examples throughout the text to illustrate how, step by step, the nurse assesses, plans and applies behaviour therapy and evaluates the effect of her intervention or of the patient's own efforts.

Attractive, simple illustrations enhance understanding. The author is scrupulous in supporting his statements with scientific evidence, but his documentation is never intrusive.

Foreword

The author points out that behavioural approaches have been shown to hold great promise for widespread problems. He deals with those of the mentally disordered, but, as he points out, all those engaged in the helping arts can benefit from each other's expertise. Nurses will find that they can apply what is learnt from this book in every field of nursing. The nurse's 'role', as described in this book, is an educational one, offering the patient the opportunity to use a range of coping skills within a carefully planned structure.

The principles of behaviour therapy are still often misunderstood, but now that this book has been published, there is no longer any excuse for this. The author has served the nursing profession well.

Professor A.T. Altschul,
Department of Nursing Studies,
University of Edinburgh

To Poppy and Charley for
shaping my behaviour and to
Albert, Boz and Mr Beckett
for the lessons painfully learned

PREFACE

Nurses help people: through birth, trauma, illness — whether short-lived or chronic — and finally through the experience of decline and death itself. They also try to help people overcome the physical and spiritual problems which stem from illness or other forms of life crisis. On occasions, however, they decided that it is more appropriate merely to alleviate distress, or to encourage the acceptance of handicaps, than to strive too resolutely for the elimination of such problems. This book has been written for nurses who see their role primarily in these 'helping' terms: offering people some kind of assistance to cope with their problems of living. At the time of writing, no clear-cut definition of the role of the psychiatric nurse, or the nurse in mental handicap, is available. However, it is clear that nurses in these two fields are struggling to remodel the nature of their activities, as well as its image. Their goal is not, I suspect, so much the regeneration of their profession, as the pursuit of an ideal of patient care. The concept of 'care' which was custodial, palliative, or even supportive, is dying fast, to be replaced by a caring concept which is positive, dynamic and resourceful. The terms 'therapist' and 'nurse therapist' appear regularly throughout the book. As I shall argue later, these titles are no more than conventions, which do not imply that the outcome of 'good therapy' is in any way different from 'good care'. This book, as the title suggests, was written for a wide audience of nurses, and is addressed specifically to those who exhibit a genuine concern for the patient, whether they wish to call themselves 'therapists' or not.

The kind of life problems which are discussed may be purely social or psychological in character. In most cases they are likely to be the psychosocial spin-off from quite different problems, such as the many varieties of mental handicap or illness. However, I have taken the view that these difficulties can best be understood in terms of 'problems of living'. Such an approach seems most fitting for nurses and certainly is most appropriate for the model which I shall describe. The kind of help which people need to resolve problems of a personal or social 'effectiveness' nature, could be called psychotherapy and those who offer such help, psychotherapists. The fact that the help offered by nurses, and often readily grasped by the patient, is not called psychotherapy, says more about the exclusive tradition of 'professional help',

1

than it does about the value of nurses as helping agents. Although there has been much debate about the status of behaviour therapy as 'one of the psychotherapies', I do not believe that we should concern ourselves with such an issue. Instead we should be concerned to evaluate the possible contribution which the behavioural approach can make to our nursing practice and to the welfare of our patients.

My reasons for writing this book were three-fold. First, I hoped that I could encourage nurses to view behaviour therapy as just another form of help-giving. The shape and form of this 'help' seems to be very amenable for adoption by nurses as another model for the presentation of nursing care. In this sense, I was concerned to clarify — perhaps in my own mind — *what* behaviour therapy is.

Secondly, I hoped that I could draw attention to the wide potential of behaviour therapy, especially since it is often narrowly described as only applicable to certain neuroses, or as a form of conditioning, suited only to children or the mentally handicapped. By clarifying the range of applications of behaviour therapy, I was concerned to say *what it is for*.

Finally, I wanted to consider the relevance of behaviour therapy to nurses in the clinical fields of mental handicap or psychiatry. The nursing process literature is trying to rehabilitate the traditional image of the nurse, as an agent of help, as well as mercy. I hope that the behavioural process described in the book will help nurses extend their therapeutic — helping — role in some small way. In that sense I wanted to say *who* behaviour therapy nursing is for, at least in the professional sense.

I have concentrated unashamedly on two strange bedfellows: the process and the ethics of behaviour therapy. I apologise, in advance, for the moments when my passion for one or the other overwhelmed me. The first two chapters set the scene for the application of the behavioural *approach*, by outlining the distinguishing features of the behavioural model and the major theories of human behaviour which have shaped its development. Chapter 3 provides an overview of the process and introduces three 'patients' who serve as models at various points in the book. Chapter 4 looks at the initial assessment, in particular the format of the preliminary interview of the patient or his representatives. In Chapter 5 a range of behavioural assessment methods is described; these are used to produce the baseline measure of the patient's problems. In Chapter 6 the design of the treatment programme is covered, from the analysis of the assessment information through to consideration of the ethics of treatment or training. The section on behaviour change techniques is split into three chapters. In Chapter 7 I discuss the techniques which operate from 'outside' of the person. In Chapter 8 the treatment methods which rely on greater patient involvement, especially in respect of 'hidden' processes — such as thought or imagination — are discussed. In Chapter 9 I discuss a range of treatment packages for the three 'model patients': these relate to group treatment, in one form or another. In Chapter 10 I review the past, present and possible future role of nurses as 'behaviour therapists', on a number of levels. Finally I review some of the issues which cropped up during the writing of this book, or which seem to be significant pointers to the future of the 'art'. A short glossary is included at the end of the book and provides brief definitions of the major technical terms used.

I should like to acknowledge the assistance I received from colleagues in the preparation of the manuscript. In particular I must thank Kate Muirhead for reviewing the draft, even when it was only in a preliminary form. I should like to thank Ian Robertson for his helpful criticism and Rob Durham for his valued judgement on parts of the text and on the concept in general. I acknowledge the contribution made by many of my students, through their enthusiasm and stimulation. Finally, I should like to thank my colleagues within the Tayside Area Clinical Psychology Department who have supported — or otherwise aided and abetted — the concept of nurse behaviour therapy.

1 INTRODUCTION

Behaviour is a mirror, in which everyone
shows his image.
— Goethe

Most of us like to think that we are the masters of our own fate, planning our every action and shrewdly exploiting the world for our own ends or for the welfare of our fellow man. The truth may be less to our liking. We may be as much the product of our environment as the masters of it. Over the past seventy-five years the social sciences have shattered various myths about the nature of man. In spite of having different standpoints, psychology, sociology and anthropology all show how we are shaped by forces in our environment. Our behaviour is influenced by genetic inheritance, but it is also determined to some extent by climate and society. The question which is still unanswered is 'to what extent?'. This question will not be answered in this book. Although some of the issues raised by the 'nature–nurture' debate will be considered, we shall concentrate upon ways of helping people change their behaviour. We shall consider ways of helping people, called mentally ill or handicapped, change their very distinctive and very debilitating patterns of behaviour.

Two avenues of help will be explored. We shall look at ways of changing behaviour from outside the person, using the power of the environment, especially other people's actions. We shall also look at ways of helping the patient engineer his own behaviour, teaching him how to control his own actions. In both cases the aim will be to build new patterns of behaviour. The end result will be a person who is more independent and less at the mercy of his environment.

The extent to which we govern ourselves is still unclear. This is due largely to the vagueness of the term 'self'. What is the self? Who are we and what are we? Such fuzziness is common to many spiritual or humanistic models of man. This vagueness may be an obstacle to increasing our understanding of our behaviour and ultimately 'ourselves'. A wide range of tools has been developed to study the physical and animal world. However, we are less objective when observing human behaviour. Even today, in the computer age, our view of our behaviour is characterised by fuzzy concepts. We continue to talk of human drives, conflicts and motives. These abstract — and unscientific

— concepts are used to explain away the mysteries of our behaviour, by implicating qualities which are supposed to be peculiar to humans. This, almost metaphysical viewpoint, is in stark contrast to the measured objectivity of botany and zoology, where the life of plants and animals is explained in more material terms. This looks suspiciously like a double standard and may speak volumes for the pompous, if not irrational, side of our nature.

The Behavioural Model

Behaviourism lays a strong claim for the title of the 'scientific approach to human behaviour'. It studies people with an objectivity similar to that practised in other sciences. It rejects concepts like needs, impulses, personality traits or strength of character as explanations of why people behave the way they do. These concepts are rejected *not* because they are wrong, but because they cannot be tested. We cannot evaluate their effect upon behaviour. The behavioural approach looks at what people do and say, to themselves as well as others. It also looks at the conditions under which they behave. Does the behaviour occur in a crowded room or deserted street? Does it happen in the morning or at night? By defining behaviour in relation to other events we are preparing to ask the all-important question: is there a significant relationship between this behaviour and these events? To what extent is the person, or his behaviour, a function of his environment?

The Interactional Model

Although the aims of the behavioural approach are simple, the process it uses may be complex. These aims are to explain, predict and control behaviour. The person is explained through his behaviour, those actions which can be measured by an observer or the patient himself. His interaction with his environment is also studied. This reveals the circumstances under which his behaviour appears or disappears, increases or diminishes. If any behaviour persists it is assumed that it is maintained by some kind of 'reinforcement'. We mix in company we enjoy and avoid people we dislike. We drink in lounge bars with soft lights and sweet music, and avoid noisy, run-down public bars or vice versa. Children work when the teacher is in class and stop when she leaves. Our behaviour is determined largely by its consequences: what happens as a result of doing this or that. Our memory of past consequences can, however, influence our expectations of what might happen if we behave the same way again. As a result, the mediating processes of thought and memory, etc., are important. Once we have identified what supports a particular pattern of behaviour, we can predict when, where and approximately how often it will occur. By manipulating the 'reinforcers' which encourage or discourage the behaviour, we can make it happen more or less often in the future. The behaviour can be brought under therapeutic control.

Behaviour therapy is concerned more with understanding the nature of man's interaction with his environment, than with the 'nature of man'. The behaviour therapist tries to explain and predict this interaction, so that a new control may be brought to bear. Behaviour therapy is often seen as nothing more than a means of controlling behaviour, implying that behaviour is not controlled already. Yet it can be argued that all behaviour is under some kind of control. Behaviour therapy merely establishes new controls which will promote a more adaptive way of living.

This interactional model is different from many traditional views of human behaviour. At one extreme people have been depicted as dependent upon their environment, puppet-like figures prodded into action by external forces. At the other lies 'autonomous Man' who is seen as wholly independent, his behaviour determined by 'free will'. The interactional model argues that people create situations in much the same way as they are 'created' by them. We are engaged in a constant process of adjustment, modifying our future behaviour on the basis of the outcome of our past behaviour. In short, we adapt to suit different, or changing, conditions — landscape conditions, weather conditions or social conditions.

Models of Illness and Handicap

So far we have discussed behaviour only in a general sense. However people who are labelled as 'mentally ill' or 'mentally handicapped' show quite specific patterns of behaviour, which is out of the ordinary: it is abnormal. People with psychiatric conditions may be described as 'mentally ill', 'psychotic' or 'neurotic'. Those with a mental handicap may be called 'mentally defective', 'subnormal', 'backward' or 'retarded'. Although these labels do not define specific conditions they suggest problems stemming from a pathological base. Labelling people as sick, ill or disabled has been seen as a sign of progress. It is not long since such people's behaviour was seen as a sign of demonic possession and was treated by a range of cruel punishments. Flogging, water torture and starvation were all designed to exorcise the demon or to render the patient's body uninhabitable by evil spirits.

The concept of 'illness' or 'handicap' has brought only a semblance of dignity to people so labelled. Although society is more sympathetic, the age-old stigma remains. The mentally ill or handicapped still evoke a negative evaluation by the general public. The same is true of the places where they are treated. Although great progress has been made, facilities for such people are persistently the 'Cinderella' of any health service. The mentally ill or handicapped are still treated as an inferior species or as a race apart.

The Medical Model

Labelling people as ill or handicapped is in the tradition of the medical model of abnormal behaviour. This assumes that deviant behaviour is a symptom of some underlying disease process. As in general medicine, treatment is aimed not at the behaviour but at the underlying problem. It is assumed that 'behavioural' treatment would bring only symptomatic relief. This viewpoint is the strongest in mental health and comes in two forms. The first invokes the basic medical approach: diagnosis is aimed at isolating the physical defect which is causing the problem, e.g. brain damage or dysfunction, biochemical disorder, etc. Treatment is physical in nature, e.g. by drugs or electro-convulsive therapy. The second version is often called the quasi-medical or 'intrapsychic' model.[1] This was first postulated by Freud, who claimed that deviant behaviour stemmed from personality or character defects or some other 'deeprooted' cause. The wide range of psychotherapeutic methods developed since Freud's time have all been concerned to promote 'insight' into these defects. There is little 'scientific' evidence to support these concepts of mental 'illness'. Few disorders have an obvious biophysical basis; those which have, Thomas Szasz[2] argues, are better regarded as physical illnesses with mental symptoms. Alternatively, the very nature of the intrapsychic approach defies 'scientific' evaluation. In mental handicap, although a number of 'syndromes' have been identified, few are treatable in the medical sense: diagnosis, as a result, often serves no more than a statistical function. In general labels may have a damaging effect. If nothing can be done, in the medical sense, the patient may be written off as a hopeless case. In this sense the medical and intrapsychic models are of limited usefulness.

Normal and Abnormal Behaviour

No behaviour is absolutely normal or abnormal. What is acceptable — even desirable — in one culture, may be grossly deviant in another. Criticism of political leaders may be encouraged in one society and lead to exile in another. Different circumstances also influence our view of the same behaviour. Undressing, making love, talking to oneself and screaming, may be acceptable in private, but may be illegal, immoral or a sign of madness if shown in public.

Our ideas about normality are shaped by four viewpoints. Behaviour can be evaluated from a *health* viewpoint: does it promote health or encourage sickness? It can also be seen as 'responsible' or 'irresponsible'. This implies a *legal* viewpoint, involving law-breaking or the infringement of some custom or convention. A *statistical* viewpoint can also be used: how common is the behaviour? Finally, we can employ a *moral* standpoint: is it good or bad? In each case the term abnormal could be replaced with the term 'deviant'. Any behaviour which is rare, unconventional or simply above or below average, is deviant. Only a value judgement can decide if it is right or wrong. To arrive at an objective judgement other factors must be taken into account. What are the class, cultural, religious or political affiliations of the person? What laws or customs govern this kind of behaviour? How does the person view his behaviour? Not least, we must take account of our own prejudices. No behaviour is ever absolutely right or wrong. It could be argued that a man, who kills himself to avoid betraying his country, has performed a noble act. We might also argue that this shows that he has lost his reason. Before labelling behaviour as abnormal we must decide in what way it is deviant. Then we must invoke a number of social, political and philosophical considerations to answer the question — 'does it really matter?'

Learning, Motivation and Individual Differences

The behavioural model distinguishes between mentally disordered and normal people only on the grounds of their different behaviour. It assumes that all behaviour is learned, whether it is adaptive or not. All behaviour shown by mentally ill or handicapped people is not abnormal. Even severely disturbed or profoundly retarded people have some adaptive skills. These have been learned in spite of any defects in their brains or biochemistry. Behaviourism argues that maladaptive behaviour is learned the same way, through the interaction of the 'person' and his environment. Any behaviour pattern — whether adaptive, like cleaning windows, or maladaptive, like smashing windows – is a function of three interrelated factors:

(1) The person's learning history.
(2) His current motivational state: the availability of factors which promote or discourage behaviour *in that person*.
(3) Individual differences: his physical make-up, intelligence, sensory-motor skills, memory, etc.

The interactional model of behaviourism does not ignore genetic or biological factors. Although we may be uncertain as to the *exact* nature and aetiology of schizophrenia, it is clear that people so diagnosed are different from the rest of us. These differences must be taken into account. All men are not born equal. Only a handful of us will win Olympic gold or split the atom. This fact is crucial in mental disorder, where people may have more than their fair share of defects. Yet we must not assume that these defects are the cause of the person's abnormal behaviour. Rather, we should ask how have they influenced previous learning and how will they affect future learning experiences?

Hereditary or biochemical structures play some part in determining the behaviour we develop. However we still need the environment in which to acquire these skills. A very few behaviours, such as smiling, appear to be programmed before birth.[3] A few others are the result of a physical defect, for example the motor movements associated with choreo-athetosis or epilepsy. All other behaviour appears to be acquired through learning. A potential Einstein or Muhammad Ali needs the right environment in which to learn his problem-solving or sporting skills.

Learning is often defined narrowly as 'education' or 'training'. However, any permanent change resulting from exposure to the environment can be called a learned behaviour. By falling on to foam rubber or concrete, we learn to distinguish the two surfaces. We can also learn vicariously, by watching someone else fall on to the same surfaces and observing the consequences. Much of our social behaviour is learned in this way. We imitate behaviour which is 'rewarded' and avoid or conceal behaviour which is punished in others. The mentally ill or handicapped appear to have learned behaviour which is ineffective or inappropriate. This has brought them into conflict with others. From another angle they appear to have failed to profit from normal learning experiences. Deficits in their behaviour repertoire make them dependent upon others. The aim of behaviour therapy is to set up new learning experiences, so that the individual can learn to be a more effective person.

What is Behaviour Therapy?

Behaviour therapy is often described as the application of the laws of learning. Writers often discuss behaviour therapy or modification in terms of classical or operant conditioning. More recently authors have emphasised the relevance of social learning theories, as an alternative to those models based mainly upon animal learning. These different theories are, however, the basis of only some behaviour-change techniques. The main feature of behaviour therapy is its experimental approach to the analysis of behaviour problems. Even in routine clinical work, therapists use a problem-solving, research-oriented, approach. This means that behaviour therapy is not an arrived-at set of procedures, based upon an arrived-at set of principles.[4] This approach emphasises the analysis of the person's interaction with his environment. From this analysis, individualised treatment plans can be devised. This will take account of individual characteristics and individual circumstances. This empirical approach means that behaviour therapy is developing continually and is not a rigid process.

In this chapter we have talked about the behavioural approach, behaviour therapy and behaviour modification. Some writers distinguish between these terms. Behaviour modification has been called the application of operant-based techniques with chronic psychiatric patients or the mentally handicapped. Behaviour therapy is often associated with other techniques, applied to less severe psychiatric problems. To complicate matters further, the term behavioural psychotherapy is often used to describe the treatment of 'neurotic' patients, yet the journal *Behavioural Psychotherapy* covers all kinds of behavioural techniques, applied to all kinds of patient groups. Behaviour therapy is used in this book to refer to an approach which emphasises the study of problem behaviour, with a view to establishing individualised treatment. I favour the term 'therapy' since this usually means 'an offer of help'. In behaviour therapy we try to resolve the problems of living of people who are labelled — usually by someone else — as mentally ill or handicapped. The term does not refer to any particular bag of tricks, used to treat particular patient groups or collections of symptoms.

The Major Characteristics

A distinguishing feature of the medical model is diagnosis of problems according to symptom categories and treatment according to pathological groups. People with similar problems might all be labelled 'schizophrenic' and would all receive much the same treatment. Although some behaviour therapists persist in using such categories to identify the kind of therapy being practised, in general the behavioural approach opposes the labelling and treatment of 'conditions'. Instead the approach stresses the need to identify and manipulate the factors which trigger or maintain problems, in particular individuals. Patients are treated as people with problems of living. These problems are acquired through learning, rather than any disease process. The major characteristics of behaviour therapy reflect this empirical, experimental, person-centred approach.

(1) Systematic assessment: all problems are defined in terms of the person's behaviour. There are three main classes of behaviour: observable acts, like walking, speaking, etc.; covert or hidden behaviour, like thinking or imagining; and involuntary behaviour, the actions of smooth muscles or glands. Where behaviour is visible it is defined through actions and their effect upon the environment. Where it is hidden, the person must define the behaviour himself. In the case of involuntary behaviour, special equipment may be needed to measure accurately responses like sweating. This assessment includes an analysis of the circumstances which encourage or discourage behaviour. These significant events may be found where, when, with whom or what the person was interacting when the behaviour was shown.

(2) Explicit treatment goals: the approach stresses the use of specific therapy targets. These are agreed before the treatment begins and are negotiated with the patient or his representative. Explicit goals define what the person should do and give him a clear target to aim for. This target is also central to the evaluation and decides whether treatment has been a success or failure.

(3) Appropriate treatment methods: the behavioural techniques selected should be appropriate to the presenting problems and the patient concerned. A wide range of methods has developed from clinical and experimental research. The therapist selects methods which are 'tried-and-tested' and which can be adapted to suit the characteristics of the individual patient.

(4) Careful evaluation: the progress of therapy is monitored from the outset. Before treatment begins the problem is measured; these

observations are repeated throughout treatment to gauge whether or not the behaviour is changing in the desired direction. The therapist may also assess the effect of different treatment or assessment methods, pieces of equipment or different therapists.

(5) Socially-significant change: it is often easy to make minor changes in behaviour, but effective therapy must produce socially-significant change, otherwise the person may be no better off than before. In general 'deviant' behaviour is socially-unacceptable behaviour. This is rarely easy to define, since it depends upon prevailing social and cultural circumstances. Behaviour therapy aims not simply to increase or decrease behaviour. Instead, the problem must be brought within 'normal limits', which may vary from one situation to the next or from one person to another. In order to decide upon these limits the therapist must compare the patient with others of his own age, social and cultural background, intelligence and perhaps even marital status and birth order.[5]

(6) Use of co-therapists: many behaviour therapists rely upon others to deliver the treatment programme. These may be nursing staff, parents, relatives, friends or colleagues. In some cases the problem may not belong exclusively to the patient, but may be a function of his interaction with these significant others. It may be necessary to change the behaviour of these other people — e.g. by training them in behavioural methods — in order to resolve the problem. Alternatively, the patient may need to learn how to change these other people, in order to maintain changes in his own behaviour.

Problems of Living

A large body of behavioural research has been established over the past twenty years. This describes the treatment of the mentally handicapped, acute and chronic psychiatric patients, the elderly, schoolchildren and other 'normal' populations such as the overweight, smokers and drinkers. In this sense behaviour therapy is egalitarian. Unlike some therapies it does not discriminate against the patient on the grounds of social class, intelligence or educational background. Through its attempts to help the intellectually subnormal and other socially disadvantaged groups, behaviour therapy has earned the title of the 'psychotherapy for the poor'.[6]

The behavioural model argues that the patient's problems are 'psychosocial' in character. Although abnormal behaviour is often seen as a symptom of disease, there are few objective criteria to support an illness model. Even where organic defects are obvious, such as with mental handicap, the person's problems are his excesses or deficits of behaviour. Although some patients' problems are only disturbing on a personal level, often we only diagnose mental disorder when the patient is disturbing to those around him. In this sense the mentally ill or handicapped may be more disturbing than disturbed. Social factors — such as employment, financial status, the ability to perform self-care skills or to co-exist peacefully with family or neighbours — lend further support to this *social* model of mental disorder. These non-medical factors are often used as the yardstick to judge whether a person needs care and protection or is ready to be discharged from it. The problems of the mentally ill or handicapped appear to be problems of living[7] based upon the person's inability to function effectively.

Problems of living can be classified under two headings: behavioural excesses or deficits. Excesses are evident when someone behaves extremely or inappropriately. A man who spends 15 minutes washing his hands, each time he visits the toilet, or who has violent outbursts each day or who talks loudly to himself when walking his dog, is showing behavioural excesses. These patterns of behaviour may complicate his daily routine, cause hostility within his family, or may so alarm his neighbours that they call in the police. Alternatively, he may be unable to behave in ways which society, or his culture, deem necessary. He may be unable to distinguish between 'ladies' and 'gents' toilets, he may lack survival or self-care skills or he may lack abilities which are important only to himself — such as being able to talk to strangers or to resist unreasonable requests. These deficits may also have different consequences. He may be arrested for the first, put into care for the second, and ignored and abused for the third. The net result is an ineffectual, institutionalised or unhappy person.

The Behaviour Change Methods

A wide range of problems of living can be helped by behaviour therapy, from basic self-care deficits to the subtleties of interpersonal behaviour. All behaviour problems can, for simplicity's sake, be classed under four headings: those related to anxiety; those which are largely a function of the social environment; those involving a lack of skill; and those influenced significantly by maladaptive thinking patterns. These crude categories may serve as a basis for discussing the major behaviour-change techniques.

Anxiety Reduction Methods.   These techniques are used to reduce specific fears or anxieties, such as fear of dogs, or anxiety-related health problems, such as tension headaches. Alternatively, the problem may involve more diffuse forms of anxiety, where the patient experiences unpleasant somatic and cognitive problems in different situations. In both cases the therapist tries to help the person behave differently in the anxiety-evoking situation.

Contingency Management Methods.   These techniques involve changing the consequences of the patient's behaviour. This may involve the reorganisation of the physical environment or manipulation of social factors, such as the delivery of 'rewards' or 'punishment'. Both strategies aim to encourage or discourage different kinds of behaviour. These consequences may be programmed by significant people in the patient's environment or by the patient himself.

Skills Training Methods.   These techniques involve structured training in the skill in which the patient is deficient. This involves a thorough analysis of the skill: describing, for example, the steps involved in putting on a shirt, holding a conversation or coping with criticism. A wide range of skills may be taught in this way, from basic survival skills to interpersonal behaviour.

Cognitive Methods.   This broad category represents the most recent acquisitions in the behaviour therapist's range of techniques. As yet they are of proven value for only a small number of problems. These techniques involve helping the patient acquire the kind of 'self-talk' or 'coping' skills which will help him overcome his learned patterns of self-defeating thoughts and will allow more adaptive behaviour patterns to be established.

These four classes suggest the possible roots of problems of living. Any problem can be a function of anxiety, the social environment, a skill deficit or dysfunctional thinking patterns. Some problems may involve two or more of these 'roots'. The first priority of any assessment is to identify the kind of problem involved; this in turn will determine the most appropriate change technique. Although certain problems — e.g. 'talking to oneself' and schizophrenia — are synonymous with certain patient groups, we must not assume that all problems are peculiar to a class of patients. For example, anxiety is most often seen in patients labelled 'neurotic' or 'anxiety states'.

Anxiety may, however, be evident in an equally disabling form, in a mentally handicapped person who is being discharged to a hostel after years in hospital. The nurse's responsibility is not to label the problem, but is to define it in terms of the patient's behaviour and the factors which appear to affect it significantly. Once this explanation is complete a decision can be made about how to resolve the problem.

The Organisation of Therapy

Many behaviour therapy reports focus upon treatment in institutions or clinics. This is largely an historical accident. Patients tend to be treated where they are currently living or in places usually seen as 'therapeutic settings'. The behavioural model is, however, committed to treatment in an *appropriate* setting, i.e. in the place which is significant in terms of the 'root' of the problem. This may not be in hospital, but could be in the patient's home, in the street, or in a public house. Here again, the behavioural model is in opposition to traditional treatment models, which often use hospitalisation as a vehicle for treatment.

However, behaviour therapy is restricted by practical considerations. If a service for mentally handicapped people is based on a hospital this will limit the practice of behaviour therapy anywhere else, with this population. We should be aware, however, that different kinds of therapy can be offered in a hospital, an out-patient clinic, or in the patient's natural environment.[8] Where possible, the situation should be chosen to expedite therapy, not as a matter of convenience. Behaviour therapy has three features which apply regardless of where treatment takes place.

(1) Behaviour therapy is always *formal*. Treatment may take place in a clinical setting, complete with consulting couch, recording devices and white-coated therapists. Alternatively, it may take place under a tree in the park, in a cafe or shopping precinct. The physical setting does not determine whether therapy is formal or informal. The nurse is committed at all times, and in all situations, to observing, directing the behaviour-change methods and evaluating their effect. This does not mean that therapy must be dull or 'stuffy'. Indeed, natural humour and a relaxed atmosphere are a helpful ingredient in most settings.

(2) The treatment programme is always *structured*. This may be clearly visible, e.g. where guidelines are provided or expressed through checklists, charts, pieces of equipment or the ordered routines of the therapeutic team. The structure may also be disguised, for example

where it is integrated into an apparently casual conversation between nurse and patient. In both situations treatment always begins with a period of assessment and is followed by a period of intervention which is monitored closely to assess the degree of change in the patient's behaviour.

(3) The treatment programme is always *goal-oriented*. When treatment goals are set, a time factor may also be incorporated. If the goal is not reached by this time some consideration must be given to reviewing the programme or to acknowledging that a successful conclusion may not be possible.

The Human Relationship

Behaviour therapy does not dismiss the importance of the nurse-patient relationship. A 'good' relationship may be of crucial importance, its presence enabling and its absence handicapping the therapeutic process. The power of such a relationship is implicit in the basic doctrine of behaviourism. The patient's behaviour is largely a function of his environment and the nurse is part of that environment. It is reasonable to expect, therefore, that the patient's behaviour will have an effect upon the nurse's behaviour as well as vice versa.

A good relationship is an essential — yet insufficient — condition for changing the patient's behaviour. The 'good therapist' must be acceptable, if not rewarding, to the patient, if she is to be effective. However, the success of therapy cannot be explained by the nurse's personality alone or by her rapport with the patient. For instance, it is well known that the nurse 'cues' particular behaviours in the patient. If appropriate treatment goals have not been set, she may cue unacceptable behaviour as easily as adaptive behaviour. This problem is common to many caring environments where positive nurse-patient relationships can have a negative outcome, by maintaining 'sick' or inappropriate behaviour.

The essential features of a good relationship are not easy to define. They may also differ from one patient to the next. Research has shown that competence and status, warmth, empathy and genuineness increase the nurse's power to influence the patient. In short, if the nurse looks as though she knows what she is doing, the patient may believe that she has the ability to help him. Her title may add further confirmation of this. If she smiles, nods appropriately and makes meaningful replies, the patient may conclude that she 'cares' about him and his problem. Without doubt, the patient's faith in the therapist is a valuable asset in any treatment setting.

Behaviour Therapy and the Nursing Process

Traditionally nursing has been seen as a set of jobs or duties, carried out by people called nurses. No real theory of nursing has been advanced until recently.[9] Since the early 1970s a major drive has been mounted to clarify nursing. Attention has also been focused upon bringing nursing under the control of a scientific, or research-based, model of practice.

Some nurses argue that nursing is not concerned with expressing the prescriptions of medical staff, but is concerned with meeting the needs of the individual patient.[10] These 'needs' may be physical, psychological or social in character. This patient-centred approach is complimentary to, but distinct from, the provision of a medical service and has been called the nursing process. The process involves the following stages:

(1) The recognition of need: the patient's problems are assessed using a rational, frequently revised, conceptual framework. Where appropriate this distinguishes between individual and normal needs.
(2) The assessment of need and possible courses of action. What needs to be done and who is best equipped to carry it out.
(3) The intervention or nursing action. In this phase the nurses carry out the nursing plan.
(4) The evaluation — the effect of the intervention is measured.
(5) The organisation and co-ordination of these four phases, including the integration of all staff involved with the patient.

This 'nursing process' is barely distinguishable from the process of behaviour therapy described. The similarities are reflected in the use of scientific method (i.e. the emphasis upon assessment, intervention and evaluation) and in the patient-centred approach common to both models. The task facing nurses in the 1980s is not to define their operation of this process, but is to define the content of their nursing action. How should nurses meet the psychological and social, as well as physical, needs of their patients? An answer to this question would help define nursing, a definition which eludes most of us.

The nursing process has become popular as a basis for the operation of nursing care. This development is helping to expedite the marriage of many aspects of the behavioural model to the nurse's more traditional role. Common ground is evident in the use of scientific method, a solid research base and a concern for the person behind the patient label. This makes nursing indistinguishable in orientation from behaviour therapy. It is too early to forecast the effect which behaviour therapy will have upon the nursing field. What is clear is that nurses are making an impact upon behaviour therapy, through provision of a service to patients who normally might be denied this facility. One would hope that the promotion of behaviour therapy is only the beginning of nurses' involvement and that this will soon give way to other contributions in the form of research and the development of clinical procedures.

Summary

The behavioural model views human behaviour largely as a function of man's interaction with the environment. This approach is concerned to explain, predict and control abnormal behaviour. Behaviourism is inclined to reject the medical or quasi-medical explanations of abnormal behaviour, suggesting instead that such behaviour is learned in much the same way as adaptive behaviour. This social model is founded upon the view that abnormal behaviour is construed as 'deviant' only after consideration of a range of social, political and philosophical issues.

Behaviour therapy is characterised by an experimental approach to the analysis of behaviour. This stresses the treatment of individuals, rather than the prescription of similar treatments to patients with the same 'conditions'. The features of behaviour therapy are: systematic assessment of problems of living and their determinants; the use of explicit treatment goals; the use of well-researched treatment methods; rigorous evaluation; the pursuit of socially-significant change; and the use of co-therapists. These features distinguish behaviour therapy from most other approaches.

Problems of living can be a function of anxiety, the physical or social environment, a lack of skill or specific thinking patterns. A wide range of treatment methods are now available, based upon these problem classes. Most of these techniques are validated by research findings from clinical practice.

The practice of behaviour therapy is always formal, with an underlying structure, and a strong goal-orientation. This approach does not neglect the positive nurse–patient relationship. This is helpful, but not effective in itself, to change behaviour.

Behaviour therapy and the nursing process have much in common: the use of the scientific method, a clinical research basis and a concern for the individual rather than patient groups. These common aims may expedite the adoption of behavioural approaches by nurses in a variety of mental illness and mental handicap settings.

Notes

1. For a discussion of the commonest behaviourist viewpoint of causative processes, read: Bandura, A. *Principles of Behaviour Modification* (New York, Holt, Rinehart and Winston, 1969).

2. Szasz, T.S. *The Myth of Mental Illness: Foundations of a Theory of Personal Conduct* (London, Paladin, 1972).

3. For an extremely important, and highly readable, account of human behaviour see: Morris, D. *Manwatching. A Field-guide to Human Behaviour* (London, Jonathan Cape, 1977).

4. This view was expressed in Craighead, W.E., Kazdin, A.E. and Mahoney, M.J. *Behaviour Modification: Principles, Issues and Applications* (Hopewell, New Jersey, Houghton and Mifflin, 1976).

5. For a more comprehensive argument read Kazdin, A.E. 'Assessing the clinical or applied importance of behaviour change through social validation', *Behaviour Modification*, vol. 1, no. 4 (1977), pp. 427–52.

6. Goldstein, A.P. *Structured Learning Therapy: Towards a Psychotherapy for the Poor* (New York and London, Academic Press, 1973).

7. The term 'problem of living' appears to have been first used by Thomas S. Szasz in his essay 'The myth of mental illness', *American Psychologist*, vol. 15 (1960), pp. 113–18.

8. Tharp, R.G. and Wetzel, R.J. *Behaviour Modification in the Natural Environment* (New York, Academic Press, 1969).

9. Scottish National Nursing and Midwifery Consultative Committee, 'A New Concept of Nursing', *Nursing Times*, Occasional Papers (8, 15 & 22 April 1976).

10. For a description see Crow, J. *The Nursing Process* (London, Macmillan Journals, 1977).

2 A BEHAVIOURAL PERSPECTIVE

We may give advice, but we can never
prompt behaviour.
                 – Duc de la Rochefoucauld (1613–80)

Most of our behaviour is learned. It is established through past experience and maintained by our present-day experiences. Once learned, it
becomes part of our behaviour *repertoire*: the stock of skills and
actions which we draw upon in different situations. As we develop we
learn new behaviour. As we add to our behaviour repertoires we
become more able to adapt to the varying circumstances of life; we
become proficient at living. If someone fails to learn the skills essential
to childhood, adolescence or adulthood, he will experience coping
difficulties. If these are severe he may be labelled 'handicapped',
'disabled' or perhaps 'inadequate'. People may also learn behaviour
which is not adaptive. Such maladaptive behaviour can cause problems
on a personal or interpersonal level and may need to be modified if
'personal effectiveness' is to be restored. Behaviour which is grossly
maladaptive may need to be unlearned altogether. In such cases, removal
of part of the person's repertoire may be to his advantage.

Many of the problems of the mentally ill or handicapped are to be
found in their behaviour repertoires. Although some 'disordered behaviour' may be the result of an organic defect, such problems are rarely
peculiar to the psychiatric population. Most of the problems of the
mentally ill or handicapped appear to have a significant 'learning'
component. Some problems may be a problem to the patient himself
or to those around him. Essential skills may not have been learned
fully or may be missing altogether. The solution to these repertoire
defects is to modify or unlearn maladaptive behaviour and to give the
patient a chance to learn new patterns of behaviour. Where someone
fails to learn how to adapt to his circumstances by natural means, then
a special kind of learning situation is clearly necessary.

The Behaviour Repertoire

Learning theorists suggest that our behaviour repertoire is composed
of three main classes of behaviour. These do not function independently of each other, but interact to produce the complex behavioural

strategies which we use to solve the problems of everyday living, or to plan for the future.

(1) Reflex Behaviour. Reflexes are involuntary, uncontrolled actions, mediated by the autonomic nervous system. These involve glands or smooth muscles and appear as responses to highly specific environmental events. Our eyes blink when irritated by dust or a draught of air; our heart rate and blood pressure rise when danger looms; we sweat when the sun is high and shiver when the temperature drops. These survival tactics are not learned: they have evolved as ways of adapting to environmental changes, and are passed on through heredity. However, some people show inappropriate reflex behaviour. When someone sweats profusely in cool weather, or blinks repeatedly in the absence of any irritant, these reflexes do not perform any survival function. Such behaviour — often called emotional — has been learned. Fear, anxiety, depressed or excited states are the commonest examples of such behaviour, where changes in heart rate, blood pressure, intestinal contractions and perspiration all may be evident. Since there is no danger, trauma or other such stimulus to account for such a reaction, such behaviour is inappropriate.

(2) Operant Behaviour. This involves behaviour which operates on the environment. Operants are maintained or eliminated by their consequences, the effect they produce within the environment. They represent a large section of our behaviour repertoire and include such diverse actions as shaking hands, undressing, building a wall, breaking a window or buying a car. Operants differ from reflexes in two ways:

(i) Operants, like reflexes, occur under certain stimulus conditions. These conditions do not, however, stimulate behaviour. Instead they 'cue' or prompt the behaviour to happen. When I see a friend in a crowd, I smile and wave to her. When given a bill in a restaurant I search through my pockets for money. When I see my friend I have a range of behavioural options open to me. I might scowl, call her name or look the other way, depending upon what happened the last time I saw her. The stimulus may 'cue' or prompt any one of a range of different behaviours. In this sense operants are often called voluntary behaviours. However, if I have not learned the appropriate behaviour — such as paying the bill — then the sight of this stimulus (the bill) will not produce bill-paying behaviour.

(ii) Operants always produce some consequence within the environment, i.e. outside of the person. Reflex behaviour produces an effect only within the person. When I smile at my friend she may smile back at me. As I search my pockets the waitress may hold out her hand. Although these consequences cannot change the behaviour which has happened already, they may influence its repetition, in similar situations, in the future. Such consequences teach us how to respond to different cues or stimuli.

(3) Covert Behaviour. This third group includes all covert, or hidden, behaviour: thinking, imagining, dreaming, hallucinating, fantasising. Although covert behaviour appears to exist in a world of its own, it plays an important part in the production of more overt patterns of behaviour. Many behaviour therapy texts define 'behaviour' narrowly, describing only reflexes and operants. This attitude is typical of the view that only observable behaviour should be studied. Since many patients in mental handicap hospitals or psychiatric clinics present problems involving covert behaviour, it would be foolhardy to exclude this class from consideration simply because we cannot see such behaviour. Certainly, we can only 'study' such behaviour in patients who can report reliably upon their thoughts, fantasies, etc. It does not follow, however, that because the patient finds it difficult to report covert behaviour, he does not engage in thinking, imagining, etc. This misguided assumption has bedevilled the field of mental handicap where uncommunicative or inarticulate patients have often been viewed as less complex than 'normal' people.

Learning

Our view of learning is often limited to the acquisition of skills and knowledge through formal education or training. Few would accept that emotions, patterns of problem-solving or social interaction are learned. The common view is that such behaviour is natural, either inherited genetically or 'willed' in some way. Behaviourism would describe any experience which leads to behaviour change as a learning experience. Although we assume that learning only comes through formal teaching, in reality we are learning most of the time we are awake. Of course, this 'life-learning' is mostly unstructured or accidental. Yet this does not prevent such experiences from having an effect upon our behaviour.

Behaviour therapy is based upon the simple truism that life is an unending learning experience. This applies whether we are aware of it or not. Our behaviour is shaped by exposure to the experiences life offers. Not everyone profits from such experience to the same extent.

Our 'individual differences' determine that some people learn quickly, whereas others appear not to learn at all. For such people 'therapy' is a new, improved — and often highly artificial — learning experience.

The Behaviourist Tradition

Down the centuries man has tried to explain himself, studying his personal experience of nature, expressed through his thoughts and emotions, and his interpersonal experience, expressed through his dealings with other men. The obvious difference between private experience and more public forms of behaviour led in some way to the assumed distinction between mind and body. Our present concept of *mind* goes back to Descartes,[1] the seventeenth-century philosopher, who proposed that all complete adults — children and the mentally disordered were excluded from his scheme — had a mind which willed the actions of the arms, legs, tongue, etc. Whenever the body smiled or grimaced this was no more than an expression of the mind's mood. Only by looking inward (introspection) could a person study his true self and find genuine explanations for his behaviour. Introspection and the concept of mind were central to the psychoanalytic movement. Led by Sigmund Freud, this group hoped to turn the study of consciousness into a serious science by defining the forces of the mind which controlled outward behaviour. These concepts are now very much part of our everyday life and language. When people lose concentration their 'mind wasn't on the job'. When we experience an emotional crisis we fear that we are 'losing our mind'. To show their disapproval of youth culture adults often describe pop music as 'mindless'. In our increasingly secular society, the mind would appear to have replaced the 'soul' as the personification of the 'self'.

Although behaviourism and psychoanalysis originated at around the same time, it was not until the 1920s that the school of behaviourism found its own strong voice. This was in the form of J.B. Watson, the American psychologist, who proposed the radical view that 'consciousness' and the concept of 'mind' were not useful subjects for the scientific study of human behaviour. He argued that such 'mental events' were no more than by-products of experience: they were the result of behaviour, rather than the cause.[2] His alternative was to study only observable behaviour, those events which could be defined and measured by scientific methods. Although he was an influential figure many found Watson's view too simplistic. It was soon recognised that thinking, image-making and other 'abstract' processes — commonly called the ghost in the machine — could be studied scientifically, as an adjunct to observable behaviour. Indeed contemporary behaviourists are giving increasing attention to the role of thinking in the production of overt behaviour. However, the study of these covert events involves much the same rigour as Watson reserved for observable behaviour and in no way marks a return to the mentalism of traditional psychotherapy.

The Learning Theories

Behaviour therapy is based upon a number of learning theories. At least three important models have been described over the last 75 years. These represent the basic foundations of most of the practices called behaviour therapy.

Classical Conditioning

Classical learning theory concerns the process by which reflex or automatic behaviour is learned. Although developed by Ivan Pavlov (1849–1936) the broad outline of conditioning theory was known long before the Russian physiologist made his exhaustive study of the processes involved. While studying salivation in dogs, Pavlov noted that some began salivating before the food was given to them. He knew that food produced salivation naturally; this was an innate or 'unlearned' mechanism. However, he did not understand why the dogs should salivate at the sight of someone who only might be bringing food. A series of experiments were set up in which various neutral stimuli (a tuning fork, bell, buzzer, light, etc.) were presented with food which the dogs ate. These stimuli were used since they had no power to produce salivation. After repeated pairings with the food (see Figure 2.1) Pavlov found that the dogs salivated when the tuning fork was sounded *without the food accompaniment*. Pavlov concluded that an association had been made between the tuning fork and the food. The neutral stimulus seemed to have acquired the power of food – the unlearned or unconditioned stimulus. Pavlov then called the tuning fork (etc.) the *conditioned stimulus* and named the response it produced a *conditioned response*. The 'associative learning' which had taken place he called *conditioning*.

Classical conditioning is relevant only to reflex behaviour. These behaviours occur involuntarily, e.g. when we flex certain muscles in reaction to pain or when we are startled. However these responses are natural. When we respond in this way to neutral stimuli – e.g. when we are startled by a photograph, or when our heart races at the sight of a

Figure 2.1: The Four Stages of Classical Conditioning

STAGE	STIMULUS	RESPONSE
1	BELL (Conditioned Stimulus–CS) ⟶	NO RESPONSE
2	FOOD (Unconditioned Stimulus–UCS) ⟶	SALIVATION (Unconditioned Response–UCR)
3	FOOD (UCS) + BELL (CS) ⟶	SALIVATION (UCR)
4	BELL (CS) ⟶	SALIVATION (Conditioned Response)

kitten — we are showing conditioned responses. The photograph or the kitten does not have any natural power to produce such reactions; therefore they must have been learned.

Pavlov's studies showed that some dogs could be conditioned quickly, whereas others took much longer. He also found that the conditioned reflex could be *extinguished*, or eliminated, by reversing the process: by repeated presentation of the tuning fork *without ever presenting the food*. Again some dogs extinguished the learned behaviour very quickly, whereas with others this took some time. It was also noted that the conditioned response often reappeared spontaneously some time later, although this was always in a weaker form than the original.

Generalisation and Discrimination. After a dog had been conditioned to respond to one stimulus, it tended to do this in response to any stimulus which sounded or looked similar. If a light had been used the dog would salivate to any light, or even something bright. This process was called *generalisation*. The dogs could also be conditioned to respond

Figure 2.2: The Classical Conditioning Model of Fear

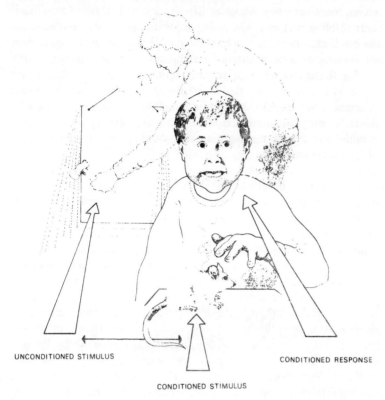

UNCONDITIONED STIMULUS

CONDITIONED RESPONSE

CONDITIONED STIMULUS

to one light and not another, by extinguishing responses to all stimuli except the one which Pavlov wished to retain. When the dog responded to one stimulus and not another, *discrimination* had taken place.

Emotional Behaviour.   The relevance of these findings to human behaviour has often been questioned. There do, however, appear to be some interesting similarities. We have noted already that 'emotional behaviour' is often associated with neutral stimuli. Fear, which usually is produced only by dangerous events, can often be stimulated by relatively harmless events or images. Many people suffer from such fears for a time, after which they fade away, often to return quite spontaneously. This is similar to the 'extinction and return' phenomenon described by Pavlov. Several researchers have conditioned emotional responses in experimental situations. The earliest example involved Albert, an eleven-month-old boy who was left to play with a white rat (Figure 2.2). After Albert and the rat had become acquainted a loud noise was sounded each time he touched the rat. The noise, an unconditioned stimulus, produced a natural 'startle reflex': Albert jumped. After pairing the sound with the rat only seven times Albert fell over and cried whenever he saw the rat. Although the noise was no longer sounded, the rat had become a conditioned stimulus, producing Albert's fear and startle response. This fear generalised to similar stimuli, with Albert showing the same reaction to wool, a rabbit, a dog and a Santa Claus mask.

Susceptibility to Conditioning.   Even if we accept the basic learning model presented by Pavlov we must ask why some people learn such emotional behaviour, whereas others appear to be unaffected by the same experience. In the 1950s Janet Taylor conditioned an eye-blinking response to light, by presenting the light along with a puff of air to the eyelid.[3] When the light was presented alone, the subjects continued to blink. Taylor found that those who had scored highly on an anxiety scale were conditioned more quickly than those with lower scores on the same scale. Although the implications of this study have been disputed, it appears that some people are more susceptible to conditioning than others. This susceptibility, which was also shown by Pavlov's dogs, may have something to do with inherited biological make-up. In short, 'temperament' may explain why some people learn emotional reactions from a single experience, whereas others require long-term exposure to achieve the same effect. Although such temperamental characteristics are in-built, this does not mean that such behaviour cannot be unlearned. The judicious use of classical learning principles may be one way of achieving this end.

Operant Conditioning

Classical learning is one kind of associative learning, concerned solely with behaviour occurring within the person. Operant conditioning is another kind of associative learning, concerned with the person's relationship to his surroundings. A large proportion of our behaviour repertoire is made up of operants; these have all been shaped by their consequences. Behaviour which generates positive consequences is 'stamped in'; behaviour producing unpleasant consequences is 'stamped out'. Although the theory was developed by B.F. Skinner[4] it is based upon the much older idea of the 'law of effect', first proposed by

Figure 2.3: Operant Behaviour in the Skinner Box

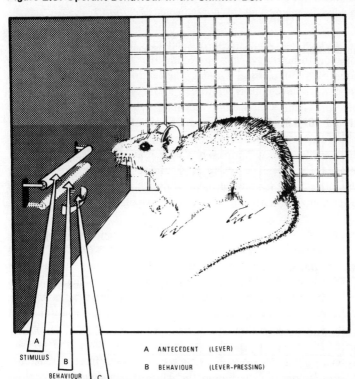

A ANTECEDENT (LEVER)

B BEHAVIOUR (LEVER-PRESSING)

C CONSEQUENCE (FOOD)

STIMULUS

BEHAVIOUR

REINFORCER

Thorndike.[5] Thorndike put cats into a box which could only be opened by working a complicated latch system. After pawing around the box the cats learned to effect their escape by trial and error. If returned to the box they would escape quicker and quicker each time. Skinner used the same kind of format by putting a hungry rat into a box which was empty except for a lever on one wall (see Figure 2.3). While exploring the box the rat pressed the lever in some way. This generated the 'consequence' of a pellet of food dropping into a dish from an automated chute attached to the wall of the box. The rat soon stopped exploring the box and spent more time pressing the lever to gain food. It had 'learned' the association between the lever (stimulus), lever-pressing (behaviour) and the appearance of food in the dish (consequence).

Since this consequence appeared to strengthen the rat's lever-pressing behaviour, Skinner called this consequence a *reinforcer*.

Reinforcement and Extinction. Although the concept of reinforcement is common to both Pavlovian and Skinnerian theories, they operate in different ways. In classical learning, the reinforcer always *precedes* the behaviour: the eyeblink is reinforced by the puff of air which accompanies the light. In operant learning, reinforcement *follows* the behaviour: it is the consequence of the action. In both cases removal of the reinforcer produces *extinction*: the behaviour diminishes in strength and fades away completely. Generalisation also occurs in operant learning. Once the rat learns to press one lever it will press anything resembling a lever. If reinforcement is given for pressing only one kind of lever, then discrimination learning will take place.

Schedules of Reinforcement. If behaviour is strengthened by delivery of reinforcement it is logical to assume that it will weaken as soon as this is withdrawn. Skinner found that this is not always the case. The speed at which extinction occurred depended upon the conditions under which the behaviour had been learned. He called these conditions *reinforcement schedules*. When the rat received food every time it pressed the lever, a continuous schedule was operating. If the food was stopped suddenly, the behaviour soon stopped. When the rat was reinforced only after a period of time had elapsed (interval schedule) or after a number of lever-presses had been performed (ratio schedule) *intermittent* schedules were in operation. Reinforcement could also be delivered at a fixed rate – after a set period of time or after a specified number of behaviours – or at a variable rate, e.g. *on average* every ten minutes or after every ten behaviours. When fixed schedules were used the rat continued lever-pressing for a short time after the reinforcement stopped. Gradually its rate of lever-pressing slowed to a stop. When variable schedules were used the rat continued pressing the lever for much longer after the food was stopped. Since this always appeared at random, the rat never 'knew' when next it would appear.

The same rules appear to apply to people. A vending machine pays out on a continuous schedule; if it doesn't we stop putting in money almost immediately. A gambling machine operates on a variable schedule; it may first pay out after a thousand lever-pulls and then may pay up twice in succession. Work behaviour is reinforced on a fixed interval. We are paid after a period of time, not according to how much work we do. If our pay does not arrive 'on time' we continue working, but not for long. Where behaviour is maintained on variable schedules it is difficult to extinguish. We appear to 'reinforce' ourselves by saying 'it must come sooner or later'.

Complex Behaviour.   Most of our behaviour involves complex actions which have little in common with lever-pressing. These examples of animal learning are only *models*; it is not suggested that human, or even animal, learning occurs only under such controlled conditions. We should also remember that although lever-pressing appears simple to us, it may be just as simple to the rat. Researchers have shown that animals can learn complex patterns of behaviour. In problem-solving experiments rats can learn complex chains of behaviour: working levers, climbing, sliding, walking planks and moving objects in a required sequence, to reach food. The parallel with human behaviour should be apparent. Dressing, cooking and driving are all complex behaviour chains. Throughout the whole chain we pick up 'cues' signalling where to go next. If we fail to discriminate the cues we end up with our buttons fastened wrongly, a burned pot or driven into a cul-de-sac. If we mis-read the cues along the chain we are denied the 'reinforcement' which awaits us on completion of the chain. If that reinforcement is highly prized we shall take more care in future to attend to these cues 'along the route'.

Positive Reinforcement, Negative Reinforcement and Punishment.   All operant behaviour is affected by its consequences. In complex actions these consequences can affect one or several parts of the overall chain. In general there are four consequence classes, each with a specific effect (see Figure 2.4). Our behaviour can result in something being *added* to the situation. For example:

(1) A man tells a joke and the people around him laugh. His behaviour results in something being added to the situation. If this encourages him to tell more jokes, we would call laughter a *positive reinforcer* (A).

(2) The man tells the same joke in different company and a woman slaps his face. Again something is added to the situation. If this consequence reduces the chance that he will tell more jokes, then this 'slap in the face' is an example of *punishment* (B).

Behaviour can also result in something being *removed* from the situation. For example:

(3) At a party people are laughing and smiling. Suddenly a man spills his drink and swears loudly. The group around him fall silent;

Figure 2.4: The Four Consequence Classes

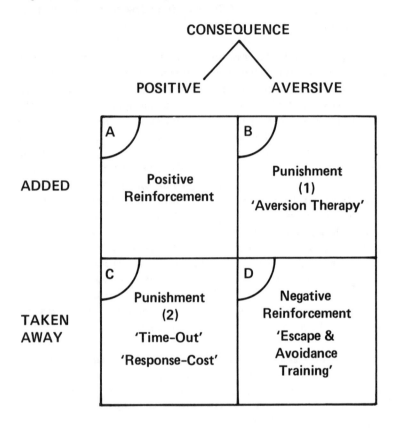

'smiling and laughing' have been taken away as a consequence of his actions. If this reduces the chances of repetition of the same behaviour in the future, this consequence functions as another kind of punishment (C). Where things are removed for a period of time, and then returned, this is called *time-out* from reinforcement. Where these are removed and never returned this is called *response-cost*.

(4) A man is watching television on a Saturday afternoon. His wife comes into the room and complains about the state of the garden. He listens for a few minutes, switches off the television and goes outside to start cutting the hedge. We may assume that the man is *escaping* from something unpleasant. His behaviour results in the removal of his wife's 'complaining'. The following week he is reading a sports magazine when he hears his wife enter the house. He rushes out into the

garden and begins trimming the roses. Here the man is showing *avoidance* behaviour: his actions prevent the occurrence of an unpleasant event. Both escape and avoidance are called *negative reinforcement* (D). In this situation behaviour is strengthened by the removal of an unpleasant event.

It has been suggested that operant behaviour is learned by one or other of these processes. It is then maintained by intermittent schedules of reinforcement. Many people would disagree, pointing out that they often do things for 'no reward' and are not forced to do them. This may be an illustration of variable or long-term reinforcement schedules. When reinforcement is distant, or appears at random, we may be unaware of the control it exercises. There may also be confusion between the technical term 'reinforcement' and the layman's idea of reward and punishment. Reinforcers may be essential elements like food and drink, or pleasurable things such as a gift or an embrace. Reinforcers need not, however, always be obvious rewards. *Anything which increases the likelihood that a behaviour will be repeated in the future is a reinforcer*. By the same token, anything which reduces the chances that a behaviour will be repeated is a *punisher*. Some children find kisses and cuddles from adults aversive and will go out of their way to avoid them. Similarly a masochist — or even a marathon runner — derives pleasure from what others might call 'sheer torture'. The simple moral of reinforcement theory is that whatever turns on behaviour in one person, may turn off behaviour in another. Reinforcers and punishers can be identified only by studying the effect of different factors upon different people. Some people are unhappy with this view, expecting behavioural theory to include a reinforcement principle which works the same magic for everyone. Yet the principle of reinforcement appears to be in keeping with the behavioural model already described. Perhaps no man is an island, but he is an individual. If we wish to study the individual, we must adapt these general principles to suit his individual characteristics.

Primary and Secondary Reinforcers.   Reinforcers may be primary (unconditioned) or secondary (conditioned). Primary reinforcers are natural: food, drink, warmth and sex, etc. Other sensory experiences might be included: the sensation of warm water which reinforces 'running a bath'; the distinctive smell which reinforces splashing cologne on our bodies; the feel of the wind in our hair and on our face which reinforces walking along a cliff-top. These are all natural: more than likely we are born liking or loathing them. Secondary reinforcers are learned. Money, certificates of merit, social approval, a new car or a painting by Van Gogh are all 'worthless' until we have learned to appreciate them. They acquire reinforcer power through association with established reinforcers. This pairing may first take place at the infant feeding stage. The mother's smiles and baby-talk are paired with food and warmth. Consequently, the mother's verbal and non-verbal behaviour becomes a secondary reinforcer. When these are paired with other 'neutral' events – like toys, possessions, etc. – these also may become secondary reinforcers.

Satiation and Deprivation.   No reinforcer is reinforcing all the time. Food is most potent when we are starving. Then we are in a state of deprivation. The reinforcer loses its power as we consume more and more of it. This is true of food, drink, sweets, cigarettes, television, exercise or sex. When we have had enough we are satiated. If we are forced to eat, drink or take exercise beyond that point, what began as a reinforcer will rapidly assume punishment status. Levels of deprivation and satiation are, like reinforcers, peculiar to the individual.

Depending upon the reinforcer involved satiation can take different forms. Too much food, drink or warmth can be both unpleasant and dangerous. The wind which began as a bracing breeze becomes painful after a time, but is unlikely to harm us. When we meet an old friend we talk feverishly for the first hour, then we begin to slow down. After two hours we start to yawn and show signs of satiation. Now it would be very reinforcing to retire to the solitude of our own room. Although too much money, possessions or conversation is rarely painful, when satiation occurs we no longer value elements which once were precious. They have become neutral or non-reinforcing.

Experimental Studies of Operant Behaviour.   One of the earliest examples of operant conditioning with people was conducted by Fuller[6] who conditioned a profoundly mentally handicapped man to raise his arm into the air. Fuller 'shaped' this behaviour in hundreds of stages, beginning with a mere twitch movement. At each movement he gave the man a small drink of sugared milk, demanding more and more movement each time before delivering the reinforcer. It is interesting to note that Itard used a similar approach with the 'wild boy of Aveyron' almost 150 years earlier.[7]

The first serious application of operant principles was by Skinner in 1953.[8] Working with psychotic patients at the Metropolitan State Hospital in Massachussets, he studied the patients in a small room, which they entered or left at will. The room contained a chair and a vending machine, which fed out sweets or cigarettes or projected coloured pictures on to a screen, whenever a button was pressed. Using various reinforcement schedules Skinner studied the subtle changes in behaviour which occurred. In this situation the only influence was the vending machine and its limited range of reinforcers. Although Skinner was not interested in changing 'psychotic' behaviour, he was pioneering an approach to the study of disordered behaviour, which led to the development of behaviour therapy as we now know it.

A notable example of the creation of an operant 'symptom' was arranged by Haughton and Ayllon.[9] They shaped up broom-carrying in a woman diagnosed as schizophrenic, using cigarettes in much the same way as Fuller had used milk. After 'thinning out' reinforcement by use of variable schedules, broom-carrying became a permanent fixture: the woman even took it to bed with her. Two unsuspecting psychiatrists were then asked to diagnose the woman. Both agreed that this behaviour was a 'typical psychotic ritual' and a function of her underlying psychopathology. Haughton and Ayllon then eliminated the 'symptom' by a rigorously controlled extinction programme.

Motivation and the Principle of Parsimony.   Apart from the ethical implications of such a project, this study raises a number of interesting questions. Was the broom-carrying a real psychotic symptom? Are psychotic behaviours learned in the same way as non-psychotic behaviours? There is no easy answer to these questions. Haughton and Ayllon were not out to dupe the psychiatrists. They wished merely to illustrate the dangers of inferring too much from the information available. One psychiatrist suggested that the behaviour was a 'magical action' . . . perhaps the sceptre of an omnipotent queen was being represented by the broom: 'She (the patient) turns inanimate objects into living creatures by cosmic forces'.[10] Neither psychiatrist ignored what he saw. However, each added symbolic interpretations which, in retrospect, appeared fanciful. Haughton and Ayllon were demonstrating the 'law of parsimony', often called Occam's razor after the fourteenth-century philosopher who formulated the principle. Parsimony suggests that a complex explanation should never be accepted where a simpler one could suffice. As Mahoney points out[11] this is only a convention. There is no logical reason why we should select the simpler of two explanations of behaviour, although in practical terms this might be to our advantage. In the example cited Occam's razor was used to trim off any unnecessary inferences about *why* the woman was engaging in this behaviour.

Skinner is a vigorous advocate of parsimony. Indeed he can be scornful of those who make inferences about behaviour which are not supported by reliable evidence. One inference which often figures in behaviour therapy is the concept of *motivation*. This was first proposed by Hull[12] who argued that a person was driven by 'needs and wants'. He argued that people engaged in behaviour to satisfy *drives*. 'Satisfaction' can be measured when the person reduces or stops showing the behaviour: his 'need' has then been met. Hull called this the *drive reduction hypothesis*; anything which reduced drive was a reinforcer.

Hull's viewpoint is commonly accepted. Most of us say that we eat to satisfy our appetite, smoke because we need a cigarette or become frustrated if we cannot satisfy our sex drive. Skinner argues that this involves making the same statement in different ways. Because we see a pattern of behaviour, we infer that it is the product of something *within* the person. In everyday life we might overhear someone say 'Mrs Smith poisoned her husband . . . Oh, how she must have *hated* him'. If we asked the person why she believed this, the probable answer would be 'well she must have hated him . . . why else would she kill him?' Of course at this level we are merely playing with words: 'murder' is real whereas 'hatred' is an abstract concept. However, as Mahoney has observed, the parsimonious view does have a practical attraction. Skinner would argue that we have enough to study by looking at how the person interacts with his environment and by considering the effect of his learning history. Examination of these elements may produce an explanation which is rooted in fact rather than shakily founded upon our fantasies. This does not mean that there is no such thing as 'motivation'. Skinner merely emphasises that an examination of behaviour, its setting and consequences, can produce a simpler explanation than one which attributes behaviour to some inferred 'need, drive or want'.

Social Learning

Evidence from classical and operant learning provides us with simple models of behaviour. One criticism of these theories involves the way in which such learning takes place. Both theories rely upon direct experience. However, it is clear that we could never build up our extensive behaviour repertoires in this way; we would hardly live long enough to acquire even basic skills. People also learn indirectly, by observing and imitating other people's behaviour. This is called *vicarious* learning; it is acquired through other people's experience.

Modelling and Vicarious Reinforcement. Observational learning involves modelling and reinforcement. A child might imitate his brother, whom he has heard swearing. The brother is the model for the behaviour, which is observed and then imitated. When a child sees his parents become anxious when confronted by a stressful situation, such as heavy debt, he may become anxious when faced with situations which are stressful to him. Fears of mice, spiders, darkness and the wind, are often passed from one member of the family to another. On a more general level the behaviour of famous people, especially film and pop stars, is imitated by their fans. When behaviour is modelled by people with 'high status' — such as a monarch, television personality or senior nurse — this may be imitated, with minor adaptations, by the 'camp followers'. Elvis Presley's 'rebellious' behaviour was imitated on a number of levels by young people, who copied his dress, hair style and way of speaking and standing. In later years these 'observers' even imitated his much-publicised religious behaviour by joining his church.

Operant learning has a commonsense ring to it. The same is true of observational learning. Many of these principles can be seen in a number of 'granny's laws'. When a child is afraid of an injection his mother will point out the 'brave' behaviour of the other boys. The child follows their example, in order to receive the praise they have been given. In observational learning, if the model is reinforced, this increases the likelihood that the observer will imitate him. If he is punished, this will reduce the chances of imitation taking place.

Classical and operant learning have often been criticised for over-simplifying man. It is often argued that learning must involve thinking and understanding. Classical and operant theory have little room for such considerations, largely because they are based upon work with animals. Skinner has argued that thinking, understanding, etc., are not relevant to the learning issue. He does not say that such processes do not exist, only that consideration of their role does not add to our appreciation of what is happening in learning. Throughout man's history, considerable emphasis has always been paid to the role of higher consciousness. In one sense, theorists like Skinner are questioning the value we attach the role of such internal events.

The Role of Mediational Processes. Learning can take place vicariously, but this does not mean simply 'by watching'. Bandura[13] lists four processes which *mediate* between the modelled behaviour and the imitation response (Figure 2.5). He suggests that the observer must *attend* to the modelled behaviour and must *retain* what he sees in order to *reproduce* the model's actions. Finally, he must have the *motivation* to copy the modelled behaviour. If the observer does not attend, there is no way that he will be able to learn the behaviour or appreciate where it would be appropriate to show this behaviour. If he cannot recall the details of the action he will be unable to 'transmit' a copy of the original. If the behaviour is beyond his capabilities, he may not attempt to imitate the model. Finally, the observer must have access to situations in which he will be reinforced for imitating this behaviour or at least *not* punished. Otherwise his 'motivation' will be low.

Figure 2.5: Social Learning — The Role of the Mediational Processes

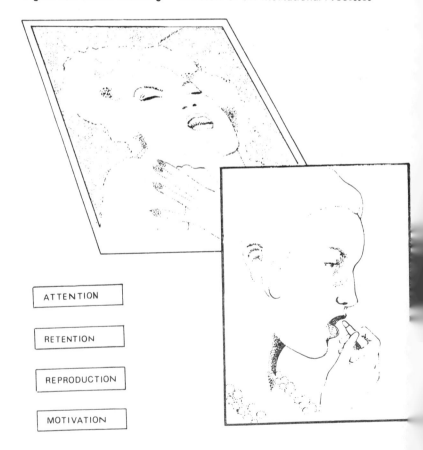

ATTENTION

RETENTION

REPRODUCTION

MOTIVATION

Observational learning involves covert *mediational processes*, links in the chain between an external event and our ultimate response to that event. These links – and our ability to use them – determine the kind of behaviour we show to the outside world.

These processes are hypothetical; we cannot prove or disprove their existence. The idea of learning assisted by such processes is not new. In the 1920s Kohler[14] studied chimpanzees who appeared to 'think' when solving problems such as building boxes or joining sticks to reach food. Others have studied rats imitating the 'successful' behaviour of other rats, during problem-solving experiments. In these situations, although mediational processes cannot be observed, the behaviour suggests that they are at work. This is not a surprising finding. It seems that few species could acquire the necessary survival skills purely by 'trial and error'.

Experimental Studies of Social Learning.   Although observational learning has been studied for many years, the key research, related to behaviour therapy, was conducted chiefly by Albert Bandura. His description of social learning[15] embraces classical and operant theory, but adds the dimension of the mediational processes. Observational learning was illustrated in two classic experiments.

In the first study[16] children were asked to play a game in which they could reward themselves with sweets whenever they wished. One group of children were shown a child playing the game who set himself very high standards, rewarding himself only when he had achieved a high score. The other group watched a child model 'low standard behaviour'. The experimenters predicted that each group would imitate the standards of their model. This was borne out when the groups set about their own games.

In the second study[17] young children were shown a film in which a child was aggressive towards a large doll, kicking and hitting it. Three groups watched different versions of the film. The first group saw the child rewarded by an adult; the second group saw him punished; and in the third film no adult appeared at all. When the children were placed in a room with a similar doll the group which had seen the model punished did not imitate his behaviour to the same extent as the other two groups. When all three groups were promised rewards if they behaved 'in the same way as the child in the film', all differences between the groups disappeared.

These studies illustrate imitative learning. It is important, however, that the model must be appropriate. This usually means being of the same age, sex, social and cultural background as the observer. If the model in the studies above had not been 'appropriate', the children would have been less likely to imitate him or learn from his experience. For instance, children of affluent parents are unlikely to model themselves on a gang from a deprived area and vice versa.

Of greater importance is the finding that learning took place on a mediational level, but was only reproduced when the model was guaranteed reinforcement – or at least no punishment. All the children in the second study learned the aggressive behaviour. However, some of them 'stored' the behaviour until the conditions were appropriate to show it.

The Interplay of Theories

Although we have discussed three distinct theories, few patterns of behaviour can be explained adequately without considering an interplay between the different models. An irrational 'fear' may have arisen through classical conditioning, but should extinguish when the person finds out that 'there is nothing to be afraid of' when the unconditioned stimulus does not appear. This behaviour must now be maintained by some other factor.

A man may become anxious whenever he sees or hears cats. This may be the result of some bad experience with cats. He may have been scratched as a child or been in an accident or taken ill, each incident involving cats in some way. His anxiety about cats may have generalised to talking about cats, pictures of cats or even being in a room where a cat has been. He may learn that escaping from cat situations or avoiding them altogether, helps reduce his anxiety or keep it at bay. We know that his anxiety should extinguish if he stays in a non-threatening cat situation long enough. However his phobia is now maintained by 'escape and avoidance' tactics which alleviate his problem or prevent it occurring.

Many people experience great fear or anxiety when there is no historical reason for such behaviour. Why are people afraid of snakes when they have never been bitten, or never seen a live snake? Why are people afraid of flying when they have never been near an airport? These phobias are not infectious, but are acquired vicariously – through watching films or television, or by listening to others relate their unpleasant experiences. In such cases the fear is learned in the way described by Bandura. Through imitation the person avoids or escapes from contact with snakes, aeroplanes, etc., in the same way as the cat-phobic above. In this situation all three models appear to be working in harmony.

Mahoney[18] suggests that the situation may involve a further dimension. The fear or anxiety shown by such patients is not a response to the *real* world. The person is, instead, responding to his *perception* of what is happening around him. An anxious airline passenger does not react to the sounds of the plane during take-off. He reacts to his perception (or labelling) of the sounds. The passenger might well be thinking '. . . My God, we've lost an engine'. Or he may anticipate (or imagine) some outcome which is wholly fictional. A compulsive hand-washer might say to himself '. . . If I don't wash my hands, God will punish me'.[19]

The investigation of such private significant events is often called cognitive behaviour modification.[20] This is the contemporary extension of the work begun by Bandura in the 1960s. The study of thoughts and beliefs adds an important dimension to the behaviourist continuum by increasing our appreciation of the range of human behaviour. It is only right and fitting that a range of theoretical models should reflect this situation.

The Behaviourist Continuum

In this chapter I have summarised the models which form the basis of the behaviour-change methods described later. These models illustrate how abnormal behaviour *may* have been learned. They also offer a framework for helping to unlearn such behaviour. All three models appear to demonstrate not only that we can give advice, but also that we can prompt behaviour.

These models are not the whole story of learning. Neither are they adequate to explain modern behaviour therapy. Many issues have been left out in pursuit of clarity. In view of their historical importance, most space has been given to classical and operant learning. However, social learning and the 'cognitive' extension appear to offer most to nurses working with the mentally ill or handicapped. Bandura's work embraces the scientific respectability popularised by Skinner, whilst widening the behavioural perspective considerably in the process.

Many behaviourists reject the model of mediational processes. Claiming to be 'radical' behaviourists they prefer to study only observable behaviour, in the manner first advocated by J.B. Watson. Mahoney believes that, although many claim to work in this way, few actually do. He believes that such 'hard-liners' are rarer than the unicorn.[21] Although critics of behaviourism often regard it as one unified movement, in reality 'behaviourism' spans a wide continuum from the professed radicals at one extreme to the cognitive-behaviourists at the other. They are all behaviourists by virtue of a common interest in behaviour and the processes which account for its existence. Although the focus of their interests may differ, they are united by the methods of scientific enquiry, which they use to build their theories or to devise a behaviour-change technology.

Although scientific rigour is essential to the laboratory or research setting, in the average clinical situation it is a pipedream. It is not possible to define, measure and control all the stimuli which may be influencing the patient's behaviour. Most behavioural programmes run on 'softer' lines. The demands of controlling even a few events while running a ward or conversing with patients is a big enough challenge for most of us. This clinical reality does not make learning theories invalid: the reverse is the case. This should make us aware of the complexity of 'natural learning'. It should sensitise us to the need to be more systematic in our attempts to arrange learning by 'unnatural means'.

Is Covert Behaviour Real Behaviour?   This chapter began with an overview of the behaviour repertoire, in terms of reflexes, operants and covert behaviour. Only social learning has room for all three classes. This does not mean, however, that the other theories rule out their existence. Pavlov considered the role of verbal and imaginal stimuli in the production of behaviour. Some of his colleagues showed that words alone could produce strong emotional reactions in people.[22] The role of language, especially in the form of self-talk, is important where the production of complex tasks are concerned. These 'private events' have become crucial components in many behaviour-change methods. Skinner himself is often misquoted on the subject of covert behaviour. Although it is often assumed that he is interested only in observable events he has said:

> No entity or process which has any *useful* or explanatory force is to be rejected on the grounds that it is subjective or mental. The data which have made it important must, however, be studied and formulated in effective ways.[23]

This is an argument against 'useless explanations', like the interpretations of the psychiatrists quoted earlier. It is, however, *for* the use of covert explanations which are supported by evidence. This must be more substantial than the product of a vivid imagination. In spite of the narrow outlook of some of his followers Skinner appears to accept covert behaviour as worthy of study: 'An adequate science of behaviour must consider events taking place within the skin of the organism.'[24]

Is Behaviour Therapy a Psychotherapy? Behaviour therapy has progressed from a stage where it considered only observable behaviour, to a situation where many therapists are eager to take account of events 'within the patient's head'. Does this mean that behaviour therapy has become just another 'mind-game'? We have discussed the concept of mind and its role in distinguishing between early behaviourism and early psychoanalysis. Some people have made a little too much of this difference. The last decade has seen a healing of the rift between the two movements: many behaviour therapists now argue that therapy means no more than 'helping people change'.[25] If we are to help people resolve complex problems of living we cannot afford to ignore techniques simply because they are not wholly 'behaviouristic'. If drugs or other methods of behaviour change make a positive contribution to therapy, it would be unethical to ignore them.

In general behaviourism is not interested in the concept of 'mind'. Skinner believes it to be an unhelpful concept: it does not increase our understanding of behaviour. However, much of our talk of mind and mentalism stems from habit, rather than conviction. Consequently the gap between behaviourism and the 'psychotherapies' may not be all that wide. It is clear that behaviour therapy is concerned with changing behaviour and not with 'healing the psyche'. However the most widely practised of all mainstream psychotherapies is supportive psychotherapy, which, along with counselling, employs techniques which are more akin to behaviour therapy than traditional 'analysis'. Viewed from this perspective, behaviour therapy becomes one of 'the psychotherapies'.[26]

When we consider the mentally handicapped, behaviour therapy looks like a godsend, mainly because so few traditional psychotherapists have shown any interest in the field. However, even here behaviour therapy is still an untapped resource. Most of the work done with the handicapped has been rigidly 'Skinnerian': the handicapped person is often treated as though he were a laboratory pigeon. My own, often unpopular, view is that the handicapped are at least as complex as 'normal' people and require access to a learning model which can explain such complex behaviour. Handicapped people can have all the problems of living which normal people may have, many of the problems of the psychiatric patient, plus a few special problems of their own. I believe that we have much to gain by looking at the 'handicapped', the 'psychotic' and the 'neurotic' as people first, and as patients a dubious second. Many of the therapeutic methods described later will have only limited application unless we adapt them to suit the individual characteristics of 'the patient'.

If nurses are committed to helping people resolve their problems of living, then they must engage in some form of 'psychotherapy'. Whether or not this is 'good' or 'effective' depends not on the theoretical model used, but upon appropriate assessment, the organisation and presentation of treatment and the behaviour of the nurse herself. The perspective of human behaviour presented in this chapter is intended for use as 'map and compass', in the exploration of problems of living. If other, more accurate and comprehensive models of human behaviour are not already available I am sure that contemporary research will soon add further, important, details to the portrait of man. The responsibility then falls to the nurse to be aware of these guiding principles of human behaviour and to use them judiciously within the context of the helping relationship.

Notes

1. See: Ryle, G. *The Concept of Mind* (London, Hutchinson's University Library, 1949).

2. Watson, J.B. *Behaviourism*, 2nd edn. (Chicago, University of Chicago Press, 1930).

3. Taylor, J.A. 'The relationship of anxiety to the conditioned eyelid response', *Journal of Experimental Psychology*, vol. 41 (1951), pp. 81-92.

4. Skinner, B.F. *Science and Human Behaviour* (New York, Macmillan, 1953).

5. Thorndike, E.L. *Animal Intelligence* (New York, Macmillan, 1911).

6. Fuller, P.R. 'Operant conditioning of a vegetative human organism', *Am. J. of Psychology*, vol. 62 (1949), pp. 587-90.

7. For a full account of Itard's work read: Lane, H. *The Wild Boy of Aveyron* (London, Granada Publishing Limited/ Paladin, 1979).

8. Skinner, B.F. *Theory and Treatment of the Psychoses* (Washington, Washington University Press, 1956).

9/10. This description of Haughton and Ayllon's study is taken from Craighead, W.E., Kazdin, A.E. and Mahoney, M.J. *Behaviour Modification: Principles, Issues and Applications* (Boston, Houghton Mifflin, 1976).

11. Mahoney, M.J. *Cognition and Behaviour Modification* (Cambridge, Mass., Ballinger, 1974).

12. Hull, C.L. *A Behaviour System* (New Haven, Conn., Yale University Press, 1952).

13. Bandura, A. 'Psychotherapy based on modeling principles'. In: A.E. Bergin and S.L. Garfield (eds), *Handbook of Psychotherapy and Behaviour Change* (New York, Wiley, 1971).

14. Kohler, W. *The Mentality of Apes*. Trans. from 2nd edn. by Ella Winter (New York, Harcourt Brace, 1925).

15. Bandura, A. *Social Learning Theory* (Englewood Cliffs, New Jersey, Prentice Hall, 1977).

16. Bandura, A. and Kupers, C.J. 'Transmission of patterns of self-reinforcement through modelling', *J. Abnormal and Social Psychol.*, vol. 69 (1964), pp. 1-9.

17. Bandura, A. and Walters, R.H. *Social Learning and Personality Development* (New York, Holt, Rinehart & Winston, 1963).

18. Mahoney, *Cognition and Behaviour Modification*, p. 5.

19. Ibid.

20. Meichenbaum, D.H. *Cognitive Behaviour Modification* (New York, Plenum Press, 1975).

21. Mahoney, *Cognition and Behaviour Modification*, p. 5.

22. Platonov, K.I. *The Word as a Physiological and Therapeutic Factor* (Moscow, Foreign Languages Press Publishing House, 1959).

23. Skinner, B.F. 'Behaviourism at 50', *Science*, vol. 140 (1963), p. 958.

24. Ibid., p. 953.

25. Kanfer, F.H. and Goldstein, A.P. *Helping People Change* (New York, Pergamon Press, 1975).

26. This view is expressed by Bloch, S. *An Introduction to the Psychotherapies* (Oxford, Oxford University Press, 1979).

3 THE PROCESS OF CHANGE

Use can almost change the stamp of nature.
— Shakespeare

In the last chapter various theories, which try to explain how behaviour is acquired, were discussed. It should not be necessary to remind the reader that even simple problems of living involve the interaction of a number of behaviours. We are rarely concerned with individual actions, such as a lever-press or eyeblink. Instead, we are concerned with the behavioural *strategies* which the patient uses: to feed himself, to express his emotions, or to make relationships. In this, and later chapters, we shall discuss ways of looking at, and attempting to modify, these behavioural strategies. For the sake of simplicity, I shall talk only of the patient's *behaviour*, meaning the flexible range of strategies he shows in response to his circumstances, rather than any concrete actions.

The 'behaviour therapist' aims to bring about a permanent change in the patient's behaviour, one which will last even after treatment is withdrawn. For some patients this may mean returning to an earlier level of functioning, behaving as they did before the problem became evident. The change may also involve 'making progress': the patient may need to learn new behaviour. In either case therapy will concentrate upon the patient's individual problems, his special abilities and the peculiar circumstances around him.

The Therapeutic Process

The final goal of therapy is to make the patient whole, to turn the *patient* (someone with a problem) into a *person* (someone with no major difficulties). Behaviour therapy has four main phases:

(1) Systematic assessment and measurement of the problem.
(2) Selection of clearly-defined goals of treatment.
(3) Changing behaviour through use of tried-and-tested methods.
(4) Evaluation of the effects of treatment.

Before discussing the techniques of behavioural assessment and therapy

Figure 3.1: The Process of Therapeutic Change

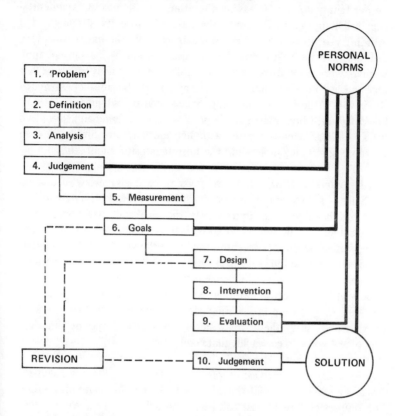

it may be helpful to draw a perspective of the therapeutic process, by considering the kind of questions which the nurse needs to ask at each stage of the programme. (An outline of the major stages of therapy is given in Figure 3.1.)

Case Illustrations

Treatment always begins with a *referral*. Here a 'problem' is identified, either by the patient himself, members of his family or some professional agency. To help study the stages of therapy the following 'cases' will be used as illustrations.

The Neurotic Patient. Mrs Smith was referred to the psychiatric clinic by her family doctor. He has been treating her mild anxiety and depression for many years. Recently, she has had difficulty sleeping and is avoiding crowds and social situations in general. She has tried various drugs with little effect. Her doctor describes her as '. . . an unhappy woman with little drive. After a childless and stormy marriage her husband left her. Mrs Smith is now staying with her mother. Although she is very critical of her mother, I believe that she is a great support to her daughter, who is making little progress towards independence.' Two weeks earlier, after a quarrel with her mother, Mrs Smith took an overdose of sleeping tablets and was hospitalised for a short time.

The Long-term Patient. Staff at a long-stay ward case review are discussing Sally — a 58-year-old woman diagnosed as Korsakoff's pyschosis — who has been very disruptive over the weekend. Night staff have complained that she refuses to go to bed. Sally also has a long history of aggressive outbursts. Recently, she broke the ward sister's spectacles, when she interrupted a quarrel between Sally and another patient. She also 'begs' for cigarettes incessantly. Staff have given up trying to reason with her because 'nothing seems to sink in'. She spends a lot of her free time dozing in an armchair, refusing to participate in ward activities. She is apathetic about her appearance and hygiene and often has to be coaxed to eat an adequate diet.

The Mentally Handicapped Adolescent. The ward sister is discussing Brian — a severely mentally handicapped 14-year-old — with his mother. She is upset because his last visit home 'turned out to be a real disaster'. She feels that she cannot cope with him 'now that he is so big and strong'. Brian is hyperactive. He roams around the ward spinning and skipping for much of his waking day. He often picks up toys and rubbish, putting them to his mouth. Although he can feed himself messily with a spoon, he often eats with his fingers. He doesn't speak, is doubly incontinent and staff say that his play skills are 'non-existent'. Although the nurses view him as a very dependent patient, they say they may have no trouble coping with him on the ward.

(1) The Problem: What is Wrong with this Person?

These illustrations are typical of referrals from community clinics or the 'continuing care' areas of psychiatry and mental handicap. Although each is different, they all imply that *excesses* or *deficits* of behaviour are interfering with the person's overall effectiveness. The patient is either behaving in a way that he finds unacceptable or is unable to behave in a particular way. In some cases that patient is quite happy with his behaviour, but others may wish that he would stop showing one behaviour or start showing another. To find out what is wrong with this person, we must ask what he is doing, or not doing, and which he — or someone else — is unhappy about. We must define his problem in terms of his behavioural excesses or deficits. Many problems will involve both excesses *and* deficits. In the treatment we may need to reduce some patterns of behaviour, increase others and perhaps teach some new skill.

Table 3.1: Examples of Performance Descriptions

Fuzzy	Performance
'Depressed'	Looks at floor during conversation. Rarely gives eye-contact. Sits bowed slightly clasping/unclasping hands. Says that she thinks 'I will never be any better than this . . . what is the point of going on. Jim left me because I was weak . . . I dragged him down.'
'Apathetic'	Sleeps in armchair during activities. Rarely initiates conversation. Speaks only in short sentences — usually these are simple requests. Pays little attention to appearance: clothing often stained, hair ruffled, buttons undone.
'Hyperactive'	Spends much of his time wandering round room (when inside) occasionally skipping or jumping up and down. Rocks back and forth in seat when obliged to sit down. Waves arms and flaps hands, stamping and shuffling his feet when seated.

(2) The Definitions: What Does the Problem Look Like?

The referrals all share another feature: they are all couched in fuzzy or ambiguous terms. Expressions like 'disruptive, depressed, aggressive or dependent' are fuzzy in the sense that they do not describe clearly what the person does. They may mean different things to different people. Two patients who are called 'dependent' or 'aggressive' may behave in quite different ways. To define the problem we must specify what the person does, says or thinks, when we (or he) think that he is 'dependent' or 'aggressive'. This will turn our 'fuzzy' into a 'performance' statement. (Table 3.1 gives examples of such 'translations'.) If problems are defined in this way the nurse, or patient, can begin to measure the severity of the problem. If they are not so defined, measurement will be difficult if not impossible.

(3) The Analysis: What is Causing or Maintaining the Problem?

Having defined what the person does, says or thinks, when the problem is evident, we now try to describe *where* and *when* the problem occurs, which *people* are likely to be present and *what* they are likely to be doing. We try to explain the problem in terms of the conditions which encourage the behaviour to appear. The nurse will try to identify the *antecedents* (what is happening around the patient, where he is, the time of day, what other people are saying or doing) and the *consequences* (what happens as a result of the patient's behaviour, what other people do or say after he has been 'aggressive' or 'burst into tears').

This analysis explains the patient's behaviour in terms of what he does and the conditions under which he does it. The concept of this *functional analysis* is borrowed from operant learning theory. However, the analysis of antecedent and consequential events in the natural environment is rarely as accurate as that which is possible in the experimental laboratory. In many cases there may be a long delay between the events which 'trigger' behaviour, and the response itself. As a result this analysis involves a value judgement. We must judge which factors have a bearing on behaviour and which do not.

(4) The Judgement: Why is this Behaviour a Problem?

Behaviourism is ethically neutral. It involves the explanation, prediction and control of behaviour. It is not about making 'good' or 'bad' changes. The nurse running the programme must ensure that change will be for the better. However, her first responsibility is to judge whether or not the behaviour constitutes a real problem. Brian's mother is very upset about his behaviour, but staff say that he is no problem. Staff in Sally's ward are most unhappy, but Sally appears quite content with her life on the ward. Behaviour problems usually involve breaking one or more of the following 'rules' or norms:

Legal Norms. Where behaviour breaks 'the law' — as in physical violence or undressing in public — it may be viewed as a criminal offence. 'Unwritten laws' may also be broken — when people 'don't do the right thing' — thereby breaking some social or cultural convention. This 'rule' may apply only to a cultural sub-group, such as a class or family group, but may be viewed as being as important as the law itself.

Statistical Norms. Behaviour which is rare is often viewed with suspicion. Where such behaviour does not infringe any legal or health norm, we must judge whether or not this problem is more than a mere eccentricity.

Moral Norms. Although most of us have values about 'good' and 'bad' behaviour, it can be difficult to gain agreement on such moral issues. Our moral outlook on certain behaviours may change significantly within generations. Not very long ago homosexuality was illegal and thought to be unhealthy, rare and immoral. Although some people still view it as immoral, we now know that it is no longer illegal, is not all that rare and is no more unhealthy than many other forms of sexual behaviour. Indeed the moral viewpoint on homosexuality is changing because of these other normative changes.

In judging the problem, we must determine which of these rules are being broken. Why is this behaviour a problem for this person? We must judge his behaviour according to what is considered 'normal' for someone of his sex, age, social and cultural background. The social behaviour of a six-year-old and a 60-year-old differ greatly. We should be aware that the social behaviour of an inner-city bricklayer and a farm labourer may also differ significantly. Behaviour problems are rarely ever absolute. Incontinence, drunkenness, swearing and talking to God are only problems if they break some norm related to age, sex or social or cultural situation, or if the patient is unhappy with his behaviour and wishes to change it. Even if these requirements are met some other moral or ethical consideration may influence the nurse's decision to treat or ignore the problem.

(5) The Measurement: How Big is the Problem?

In the last stage of assessment the problem is measured. How often or for how long does he show the behaviour? In some cases the patient may measure his own behaviour. In other settings the problem may be measured in terms of how staff or relatives 'see' the problem. The measure selected depends upon the nature of the problem. 'Hitting people' or 'wetting the bed' could be measured in terms of how often they happen each day. Other behaviours — like eating, sleeping or talking — might be measured in terms of *time spent* in the behaviour. At the end of this stage we should know:

(1) What the problem is.
(2) The conditions under which it occurs.

Figure 3.2: Presentation of the Baseline Data

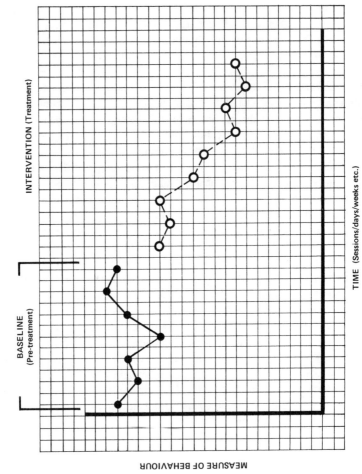

(3) Why it is a problem.
(4) How big a problem it is at present.

The measures taken in this last stage describe the problem before treatment; this is usually called the *baseline*. These measures are often put on a graph so that we can evaluate the problem: is it reducing, growing bigger or remaining unchanged? (See Figure 3.2.)

(6) The Goals: What Kind of Behaviour Should the Person Aim For?

Treatment is aimed at increasing some patterns of behaviour and decreasing others. We might want to increase the time Mrs Smith spends in crowds, to decrease the number of times Sally asks for a cigarette or to increase the number of times Brian uses the toilet and to decrease the number of times he wets himself. Each of the cases described has several problems. These would be ranked in order of priority (see Table 3.2) and then the nurse would try to decide how these goals should best be reached.

Each of the targets listed on the table represents a final goal. This defines how the patient should behave at the end of treatment. It is unrealistic, however, to expect the patient to change overnight. Instead of aiming directly for these final goals a number of sub-goals are set. Each of these becomes progressively more difficult as the programme

Table 3.2: List of Possible Final Targets

Mrs Smith	1. Increase assertive skills.
	2. Decrease anxiety in social situations.
	3. Increase time spent in crowds.
	4. Increase positive self-talk behaviour.
	5. Increase time asleep at night.
Sally	1. Decrease frequency of aggressive outbursts.
	2. Decrease frequency of inappropriate cigarette-begging.
	3. Increase frequency of washing and grooming.
	4. Increase time spent in social activities.
	5. Increase independent eating.
Brian	1. Reduce frequency of daytime incontinence.
	2. Increase time spent sitting appropriately.
	3. Increase time spent in simple play activities.
	4. Decrease frequency of 'emotional outbursts'.
	5. Increase appropriate cutlery use at meals.

Figure 3.3: The Stepladder Route to the Final Goal

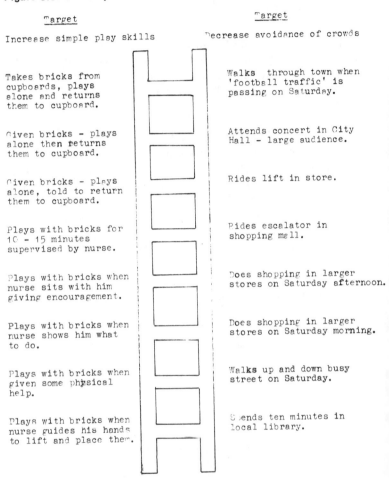

Target

Increase simple play skills

Takes bricks from cupboards, plays alone and returns them to cupboard.

Given bricks - plays alone then returns them to cupboard.

Given bricks - plays alone, told to return them to cupboard.

Plays with bricks for 10 - 15 minutes supervised by nurse.

Plays with bricks when nurse sits with him giving encouragement.

Plays with bricks when nurse shows him what to do.

Plays with bricks when given some physical help.

Plays with bricks when nurse guides his hands to lift and place them.

Target

Decrease avoidance of crowds

Walks through town when 'football traffic' is passing on Saturday.

Attends concert in City Hall - large audience.

Rides lift in store.

Rides escalator in shopping mall.

Does shopping in larger stores on Saturday afternoon.

Does shopping in larger stores on Saturday morning.

Walks up and down busy street on Saturday.

Spends ten minutes in local library.

moves closer to the final goal. Figure 3.3 illustrates the 'stepladder' route to the final goal.

Goals are decided upon according to the characteristics of the individual patient. The final goal for Brian's incontinence might be to 'use the toilet appropriately when taken by nurse or mother'. For another patient the goal might be to 'use the toilet independently'. Mrs Smith should be able to decide upon her own goals. In Brian and Sally's case a decision may need to be taken collectively between staff and parents or relatives.

(7) The Design: How Will the Person Achieve These Goals?

The treatment programme is based upon the information collected during the assessment. This provides the basis for selecting therapeutic techniques which have been effective with problems of a similar nature. The treatment programme must also acknowledge the resources available in terms of time, staff and expertise.

Information. In the assessment the nurse will have studied the conditions under which the behaviour occurred. To design the programme she must ask herself, 'Does the behaviour . . .

   . . . only happen in certain places?
   . . . only happen at certain times of day?
   . . . only involve certain people?
   . . . involve the use of any materials or part of the environment?

There is no point in arranging treatment to take place in 'insignificant' situations, where the problem is unlikely to show itself.

Techniques. Behaviour therapy prides itself upon its use of research findings. These show which techniques are effective in changing particular patterns of behaviour. The nurse must select techniques which have the best chance of success with the problems concerned. However, before making her choice she must decide upon the general nature of the problem. At a very basic level most problems can be divided into two classes: skill or motivational deficits. In a skill deficit the person could not perform the behaviour, even if his life depended upon it. Brian could not use the toilet, build blocks or use a knife and fork; he does not have the necessary skills. On a subtler level Mrs Smith may be unable to tell her mother to stop running her life – without bursting into tears. In both cases the patient needs to learn new patterns of behaviour. This may involve expanding existing skills or 'starting from scratch'. Where the problem is a motivational deficit the patient *could* behave in this way, but chooses to do otherwise. Brian can use a spoon, but rarely does so. Mrs Smith can go into shops and ride an escalator, but often decides that it is not worth the upset. In these cases the patient must be helped to show the behaviour which is already part of his repertoire, by trying to ensure that it 'pays off' in a positive way or does not have aversive consequences.

    Behavioural techniques can be subdivided unto two crude categories: those which teach new skills and those which motivate the patient.

Resources. It is easy to design an ideal treatment programme. It is more difficult to prepare one which takes account of the resources available. The nurse must ask:

(1) How much time will be needed to run the programme?
(2) Will the support of other nurses, relatives or patients be needed to run the programme?
(3) Are any special pieces of equipment needed?
(4) How experienced am I, or the other nurses involved, in using these behaviour-change techniques?

An appropriate treatment programme must take account of these questions. If it does not, the programme may begin, but is unlikely to succeed. In general, it is advisable to devise a programme which uses a small number of *familiar* treatment methods which can be handled easily by available staff, rather than relying upon a range of unfamiliar techniques which may confuse or tax the team.

(8) The Intervention: How Will the Programme be Operated?

The immediate questions to be asked at this stage are:

(1) Who will run the programme?
(2) Is there need for a supervisor?
(3) Is there need for special training of any staff member?
(4) How will the programme be monitored?
(5) Will the programme run as part of routine duties?

The 'Therapist'. The first decision must be to appoint the 'central therapist'. This person will co-ordinate the programme. In Mrs Smith's case this might be a community psychiatric nurse, who could see her at an out-patient clinic, could accompany her in town or run sessions in her own home. Mrs Smith's mother might be recruited as a 'co-therapist' if appropriate. In hospital the nursing team might present the programme, supervised by the nurse-in-charge or a clinical nurse specialist. Brian's mother and Sally's fellow patients might also have a significant role as co-therapists.

Supervision. So far we have talked only of therapy designed and delivered by nurses. Where a body of experience in behaviour therapy exists, an appropriate nursing supervisor should be available. Where nurses do not have enough experience to design or run the programme independently a supervisor from another profession may be required (e.g. a clinical psychologist). This arrangement would not remove the nurses' responsibility for their part in the programme, but would allow the supervisor to co-ordinate treatment. This involves *delegation* (deciding who is capable of doing what) and *troubleshooting* (resolving any technical or administrative problems as soon as they emerge).

Training Needs. The supervisor must question the ability of 'front-line' staff to carry out the programme. Do they need training, advice or close supervision, to carry out the programme efficiently and effectively? Even where behavioural methods are used routinely, consideration should be given to the need for further training. Does the nurse know how to use particular assessment or treatment methods? Does she know how to complete the evaluation records? Does she know what to do with these records once they have been completed? Does she know who to ask for advice? Even where staff are very experienced there may be a need for 'topping up' of skills and knowledge, through discussions, workshops and seminars. In all situations there should be an opportunity to meet and discuss the programme. Where the nurse works alone she should take time to question her own capabilities, in much the same way as she would assess the expertise of junior staff.

Monitoring Progress. A suitable recording format should be devised before the programme begins. This will be used to evaluate the treatment's effects. This fulfils a similar function to blood pressure or temperature charts. This record will show whether or not the patient's behaviour is changing in the desired direction. The kind of record used depends upon the nature of the problem, the treatment situation and the characteristics of the patient. Mrs Smith may be able to monitor her own progress through 'diary reports' which the nurse will help her analyse each week. Staff working with Brian or Sally might use a checklist, supplemented by written comments, to record what happens each time they operate the programme.

Any evaluation record must be both simple and inclusive. It must not be so complicated or time-consuming that staff, or the patient, avoid using it. Neither must it be so simple that it fails to reflect the important aspects of the treatment programme.

Routine or Special Treatment. A decision must be taken to arrange treatment within the patient's routine day, or as a special extra. Many problems can only be solved in the situation in which they arise — in the natural environment. There may be an advantage, however, in arranging special sessions to complement, or to prepare the patient for, real-life exposure. A child who is learning to eat with a spoon may benefit from extra 'spoon-use' sessions. An anxious patient may benefit from clinic-based sessions, where he can rehearse coping with anxiety in specific situations.

(9) The Evaluation: Are the Goals of Therapy Being Achieved?

If the recording format is reliable it should be an easy matter to judge whether or not the goals of treatment are being reached. Since the goals are explicit – in terms of doing more or less behaviour – it should be clear whether or not this is happening. A simple graph will show whether Mrs Smith is spending more time in crowds, whether Sally is asking less for cigarettes or if Brian is wetting more or less frequently. In all cases therapy involves trying to make the patient 'happier', 'more confident' or less 'emotionally disturbed'. We can judge whether or not this is happening by assessing the increases or decreases in behaviour.

(10) The Last Judgement: Behaviour-change or Programme-change?

The last question in the process has three facets. If the programme has changed the patient in the direction intended, is it now time to think of ways of phasing out the treatment? If the goals have not been reached, what can be done to revise the programme, so that they may be achieved second time around? In some cases the programme may have been revised several times already, in an attempt to correct its deficiencies. If the goals still are not being reached, it may be necessary to admit defeat. This need not mean abandoning the patient, only giving up on a particular treatment approach. Other approaches – or 'therapists' – may be able to help the patient where behaviour therapy, or the therapists involved, have failed.

Summary

The behavioural process illustrated shows how much time needs to be devoted to assessment and planning before we can begin to change behaviour. The process also shows how the whole programme relies upon the personal norms of the patient; these indicate whether or not there is a problem, whether the goals of therapy are reasonable, and when they have been reached. This process provides a framework for looking at the patient's problems more objectively. The nurse's relationship with the patient is sub-divided into separate units, each one making it clear what she is doing and why.

The organisation of treatment along the lines indicated should also afford some benefits for the patient. He should gain:

(1) A clear idea of what is his problem, in terms of behaviour.
(2) An understanding of the treatment methods used.
(3) A clear appreciation of his rate of progress.
(4) An awareness of the events which have been maintaining his problem.
(5) A clear understanding of his relationship with the nurse.

The process of therapy can be a convoluted trail, with a number of dead ends and false signposts along the route. The stages outlined in this chapter provide the nurse with some idea of where she is going, and where she should return to, if things go wrong. This simple organisational framework should help her demonstrate that the patient can change patterns of behaviour which often appear to be stamped, indelibly, by nature.

4 ASSESSMENT: IDENTIFYING THE PROBLEM

The greatest deception men suffer is their own opinions.
— Leonardo da Vinci

Behaviour therapy is about changing behaviour. It is not about *curing* or otherwise altering, mental illness or handicap. This *idiographic*, or person-centred approach, involves the study of a unique individual. Treatment is designed to suit this one person and perhaps no other. Traditionally, we have emphasised the similarities between patients. Often, this leads to the prescription of standardised treatment. Since nurses are more concerned with problems of living than diagnoses, they must study the person who experiences the problem, if they are to help the patient. Of course, I am not suggesting that diagnoses should be ignored. However, where it serves little more than a labelling function, the nurse must question the relevance of the diagnosis to the nursing plan.

Why Assessment?

The nurse's first goal is to identify the patient's problem. The assessment may be a complex affair, involving study of the person on a number of levels. Rigorous assessment is necessary for two reasons. First, we need to reveal the nature of the problem: defining what the person does, says or thinks (which is problematic) and describing how this affects events in his life and how he is affected in turn. Secondly, we must ensure that we pick the most important behaviour as the target for change. The patient rarely has only one problem. Assessment involves putting these various problems into perspective. We try to ask 'Why is this a problem for this person? If it is not a problem now, is it likely to become one in the future?' In this sense, assessment is concerned with *potential* problems, as well as those in the 'here and now'.

The Whole Man

This chapter is headed by a quotation and includes a famous image (Figure 4.1) both from the hand of Leonardo da Vinci. His image of the ideal proportions of man is an apt illustration for a chapter on

60

assessment. In *holistic* assessment the person is studied as an integrated whole, rather than as a collection of disconnected parts. Da Vinci would never have measured or described a hand without relating it in size, shape and function to other parts of the body. Measurement of an individual unit is of little value without the perspective of the whole. A record of 'temper outbursts', an 'anxiety' rating or description of an obsessional ritual must be seen against the backdrop of the person's overall behaviour. The assessment must paint in the background to

Figure 4.1: Assessing the Whole Person

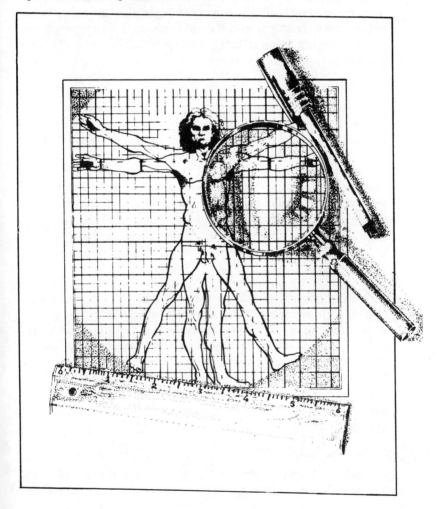

these problems: it must include his other difficulties and his assets or good points.

Traditional psychiatric diagnosis has a double-edged weakness. The concept of a problem is based upon our value-judgements. Physical health can be defined in terms of the absence of any structural or functional abnormalities. Apart from *medical* syndromes or diseases (e.g. Down's syndrome or Huntington's chorea) most definitions of mental illness or handicap are nowhere as precise as their medical equivalents. Secondly, psychiatric diagnosis looks at what is wrong with the person, rarely taking account of his assets. Behavioural assessment tries to avoid making too many value judgements, considering the patient's assets and his deficits. If the patient's assets can be strengthened, the 'person' will be strengthened. Making the person more effective is one way of tackling his problems of living.

The Assessment Process

The nurse's aims in assessment are to describe the patient's problem within the context of the whole person, to analyse its nature and function and to produce a measure which will help in evaluating change across time (see Figure 4.2). The assessment process is a chain of stages which involves 'taking pictures' of the patient and his problem. A different quality of picture is produced at each stage. At the first interview our image is crude and may be inaccurate in parts. By the time we reach the end of the baseline our picture should be like a good quality snapshot.

The Preliminary Interview

In the first interview the nurse prepares the ground for a closer analysis of the patient's problem. At the same time she establishes a therapeutic or 'working' relationship with the patient or the 'significant others' involved in his care. Her first aim is to take a simple history. Most of the first interview will be devoted to this end. An example of a typical interview schedule is given in Appendix 1. This is used to summarise notes taken at the interviews. Information from a number of interviews can be kept neatly in one booklet and stored safely in the patient's case file.

Interviewing Techniques

Interview skills are complex and beyond the scope of this book. However the following guidelines might help the novice avoid major pitfalls.

Figure 4.2: Developing a Picture of the Patient

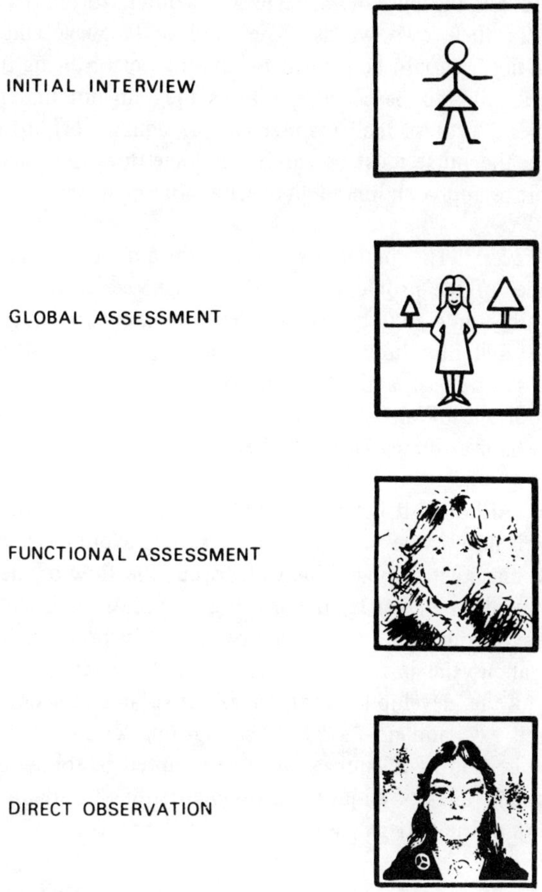

INITIAL INTERVIEW

GLOBAL ASSESSMENT

FUNCTIONAL ASSESSMENT

DIRECT OBSERVATION

The Setting. Interviews should always take place in private. This rule should apply even where other nurses are being interviewed about patients in their care. Where an interview room is not available, care should be taken to avoid interruptions and distractions. The major consideration should be to put the interviewee at ease and to give a clear impression that any comments made will be treated with the strictest confidence.

The Opening Gambit. An explanation should be given as to *why* the interview is taking place and how the nurse hopes it will develop. Although the nurse may have some details about the problem already, she should ask the patient, or significant other, to tell her about the problem 'in their own words'. The kind of language and degree of formality used, should be gauged to suit the person being questioned. Few people like to be asked questions they do not understand. An icily-efficient 'professional' manner can be equally offputting. At the same time the nurse must be careful that she does not 'talk down' to the patient or approach him in an over-familiar manner.

Ground Rules.   The patient, or other, should be asked to give his 'experience' of the problem. The nurse might set other ground rules to help allay any anxiety about what the interview might involve. She might tell him how long she expects it to last, what kind of questions she will ask and what kind of answers she hopes he will give. Most important of all, she must make it clear that she is there to listen to whatever the patient, or other, has to say.

The Plan.   Although it is helpful to have a rough plan of the key questions which have to be asked, the nurse should avoid restricting herself to a rigid checklist format. This will disrupt the flow of the conversation and may hinder her from following up points not included on her original list. A question often asked by nurses is 'how much do I need to know about the patient?' The answer is *'everything* . . . which is relevant to the development of an effective and efficient treatment programme . . . and no more!'[1] The warning 'enough but no more' should be heeded by all nurses who are tempted to follow interesting, but irrelevant, lines of enquiry. In psychiatry this invariably means an exploration of the patient's sex life.

Reflection.   In order to encourage the patient to expand upon important points, the nurse should 'reflect' − or bounce back − certain answers. The nurse re-states what the patient has just said, giving emphasis to what she considers to be significant comments. For instance, 'I see . . . you are on edge *all the time* . . . the children *react badly* to this . . .' (pause). The pause allows the patient, or other, to expand upon what was meant by 'on edge all the time' and 'react badly'. If the patient does not follow this up − or goes off at a tangent − then more direct questioning may be required. In most cases the questions used should be 'open-ended'; this means that they cannot be answered by 'yes or no'. The nurse would ask questions like 'tell me how you *feel* about . . .; what do you *think* about . . . etc.' The nurse should take care to avoid putting words into the patient's mouth, e.g. by 'suggesting' that the patient feels this or that or that he has one problem or another.

Redefining the Problem. After the patient has given a general overview of his situation the nurse should try to define the key points more clearly. The nurse is aiming for a more specific description of what the patient says, does or thinks. Once again, the nurse will 'reflect' comments made during the interview, this time asking the patient to give a little more detail about what he meant by 'being uptight' or 'at the end of my tether'.

The Conclusion. The nurse should summarise the points which have been discussed, giving her 'judgement' of the problem as a concluding statement. She should encourage the patient to correct this view where appropriate. A date should be set for the next interview and an idea given of what it will entail. Finally, it may be helpful to give a simple assignment, to complete for the next meeting. The patient might be asked to make some 'diary notes' about the problem, or care staff could keep a record of some aspect of the patient's behaviour, as they see it on the ward.

It is important that the term 'interview' is not interpreted too narrowly. An interview, taken during a walk around the hospital grounds, may yield more information than one taken in the austere surroundings of a psychiatric clinic. The information collected depends more on the interviewer's behaviour, than on the physical surroundings. However a 'good' interviewer will always try to pick an appropriate setting for the patient concerned.

Rules about note-taking are equally flexible. A tape-recorder can be a valuable aid, releasing the nurse's full attention to her line of questioning. Alternatively she may make notes on key points, as they occur, re-writing these in full once the interview is over. The golden rule is never to rely upon memory for too long. Emphasis may be given to aspects of the case which do not merit it and important details may be forgotten.

Interviewing the Patient or 'Significant Other'

In formulating the history the nurse must decide, in advance, who she is going to interview. The interview may be limited to the patient alone, where he can give all the necessary information. Occasionally it may be helpful to supplement this by discussing the problem with 'significant others', especially his family and any care staff involved. Where the patient is uncommunicative, the nurse must rely entirely on the views of his family or the nurses who come into contact with him on the ward.

Taking the History. The first page of the interview schedule (Appendix 1) is used to make notes about the patient's medical and personal history. Does he have a specific medical condition? When was it first diagnosed? Does he have any specific handicaps? When was he last examined medically? What was the outcome and what is his current medical treatment? These 'medical' factors may have a strong bearing on the 'referred problem' and must be taken into account. Most of this information can be drawn from existing records and the nurse should familiarise herself with the details before checking them with the patient, or other, in the interview.

Details about the patient's personal history can be noted at various stages during the interview and need not be pursued through a rigid line of questioning. However the nurse will want to know:

- Does the patient have a job? Where does he work and what does he do? Did he ever work? How long ago?
- Does he have a family? What does it consist of? Does he keep in close contact? Where do they live – in what kind of neighbourhood?

As we noted earlier, class and cultural values play a part in deciding whether behaviour is acceptable or not. These sorts of questions will reveal the patient's class or cultural background in very broad terms. This information will be helpful when the nurse tries to establish *why* the problem is a problem for this patient. She will also want to know something of his habits:

- What is his appetite like? What does he enjoy eating and where? Has his appetite been upset recently?
- Does he go to bed early or late? Does he waken during the night or early in the morning? Does he ever have nightmares? Does he have trouble getting off to sleep? Has his sleep pattern been upset recently?
- Does the patient go out often? Where does he go and with whom? What sort of social activities does he enjoy? Has his social behaviour changed at all recently?
- Is the patient married, single or divorced? Does he have a stable relationship at present? When did he last have a relationship?

Is he heterosexual, homosexual or celibate? Has his sexual relationship been upset of late? In what way?

Eating, sleeping, social and sexual behaviour are studied because they may tell us a lot about the patient's survival and civilised habits. Also, if the patient is experiencing severe problems in one area of behaviour, this may have some effect upon these routine patterns of behaviour. These questions need not be pursued in a formal manner, but may be picked up at points during the conversation. Questioning about sexual behaviour may be a touchy subject for some patients — and indeed for some nurses — and should be handled with appropriate respect and diplomacy.

Our thumbnail sketch is completed by noting down the patient's assets and deficits. What does he gain recognition or approval for doing? What is he proud of about himself? Alternatively, what are his major deficiencies? What changes in his way of living would he find to his advantage? If discussion about the patient's major problem has not already taken place, this question will provide a suitable introduction.

In this first interview the nurse tries to judge what the referred problem *means*, in terms of problems of living. To what extent does it break cultural norms? In what way is it upsetting to the patient? At the end of the interview the nurse should write a brief description of the problem, based upon her evaluation of the information provided. She should make a note of any aspect of the patient's behaviour which does not fit the categories listed, under the heading 'general observations'.

The Global Assessment

In the global assessment the nurse tries to add more general information to the picture of the patient's behaviour. This can best be done by using some kind of rating scale or questionnaire. These standardised assessments provide more detail about the patient's strengths or weaknesses and help decide which areas of behaviour merit closer study. It is not possible to describe the kinds of global assessments available or how they are used. However, a brief description of some of the more popular scales and questionnaires is given in Appendix 2.

Some people would dispute the need for global assessment, arguing that the 'referred problem' is *the* problem. Although this may be true there is no harm in checking that other, perhaps more important problems, are not hidden in the background. If we look at the cases described in the last chapter, we might find that each patient had problems other than those referred.

Mrs Smith presented with a simple case of 'agoraphobia' — or did she? An anxiety rating scale might show that she experienced 'fear and tension' in a number of situations. However, closer study might show that she was most anxious in *social* situations. An 'assertion' or 'social skills' scale might shine more light on this area: assessing how she copes with everyday social life and handles awkward situations or people who are 'being difficult'. After applying these measures we might want to change our original judgement. Perhaps Mrs Smith's problem is not simply a case of excessive anxiety, but is more a *deficit* of social or coping skills, which lead to anxiety.

Sally, who was causing trouble on the long-term ward, might also benefit from a wider-ranging assessment. The original judgement suggested that the problem was an excess of aggressive or disruptive behaviour. Rating scales could be used to describe her everyday behaviour, her self-care skills and social and recreational activities. The nurses might wish to consider the extent to which Sally's maladaptive behaviour is related to a *lack* of appropriate social and recreational skills. In view of her diagnosis of Korsakoff's psychosis, it might be helpful to have a specific assessment of memory and cognition, carried out by the clinical psychologist, to decide what effect problems in these areas might have upon the disturbed behaviour first referred.

The same broad assessment may help explain Brian's problems. Like Sally, he may spend a lot of time being 'disruptive' because of a lack of more appropriate patterns of behaviour. Again, rating scales of self-care and social skills will provide an overview of deficiencies in these areas. These may be as important as the excesses which led to the original referral.

The global assessment may be done as a separate exercise or as part of an interview. Care staff may be asked to complete a scale as part of their routine observation of the patient and to report back at the next interview. The patient may be given a scale to complete as a 'homework assignment' from the second interview, after the nurse has explained the use of the scale and demonstrated the method of completing it. Alternatively, the nurse may complete a scale or questionnaire in the second interview, by asking the patient, or other, the questions or by sitting with the person as they complete it. Care should be taken not to inconvenience the patient, or other, by asking them to complete such scales when they are busy, or within too short a time. The nurse must also be selective about the kind of scales to give to staff or patient and relatives. Those designed for staff may be wholly inappropriate for people who have no special training and can lead to confusion. However, by the end of this second phase the nurse should have a clear idea of all the patient's major problems and can proceed to study these in more detail in the functional analysis.

The Functional Analysis

If the assessment identifies more than one problem, then these should be ranked in some order of priority and analysed separately. The functional analysis described below is drawn from the work of Kanfer and Saslow[2] who suggested that behavioural assessment involved the following steps:

The analysis of the problem situation. Problems are defined as *excesses* or *deficits* and a brief description of their frequency, and appropriateness, is noted along with the conditions under which the problem occurs.

The clarification of the problem. Details about the 'significant' people, situations and events, associated with the problem are added.

The motivational analysis. The people, events and objects, which appear to promote or discourage patterns of behaviour in the patient.

The developmental analysis. The patient's development is described briefly. These 'personal norms' help decide why this is a problem for this patient.

Analysis of self-control. The extent to which the patient uses 'self-controlling' behaviour. If such skills are not evident, drugs and careful supervision may be necessary.

The analysis of social relationships. Details are made of the significant others in the patient's social network and his relationship with them.

Analysis of social–cultural environment. This step takes account of the norms expressed by the laws and social conventions of the patient's society, especially where they differ from his own 'personal norms'.

The Problem History

The first two stages of the functional analysis are the problem history and analysis. The nurse already has some details about the origins of the problem, from the first interview. These points are followed up in greater detail and noted on the appropriate part of the interview schedule (see Appendix 1).

The Description.   The nurse re-states the description of the problem given earlier and asks if it has changed in any way. The description can be left in a 'fuzzy' or subjective state at this stage; by the end of the interview the description should be clearer and more objective.

Previous Therapy.   The nurse will want to know what kind of measures have been tried so far, to manage the problem. How successful have they been? Are they still being used, and if not, why were they stopped?

Frequency.   How often does the problem occur, each hour, day, week etc.?

Intensity.   Is the problem becoming worse, slightly better, or is it just the same as it was last month, year etc.?

Duration.   Does it last for a specific period of time? If so, how long?

Location.   Does it only happen in particular places?

Persons.   Are any particular people usually present when the problem occurs? Who are they and what is their relationship with the patient?

Situations.   Does the problem occur at a particular time of the day or night? Does it occur during any activity or when the patient is engaged in some private activity? Does it ever happen when the patient is preparing for, or returning from, some activity or event?

Materials.   Does the patient make use of any material object, or aspect of the environment, when performing the behaviour?

Norms.   The problem must be seen as abnormal by someone, otherwise it would not have been referred for treatment. The nurse must clarify which norms – or rules – are being broken by the offending behaviour. The nurse tries to find out if this is a problem for the patient (personal), his family or friends (cultural) or society at large (social). A problem like 'drunkenness' might break all three norms, whereas 'anxiety' or 'obsessional thoughts' are only problems on a personal level. Alternatively, 'aggression' may be acceptable to the person showing the behaviour, but may be wholly unacceptable on a cultural or social level.

Defining 'norms' can be a difficult exercise. Psychiatric diagnosis often takes a more absolute view of maladaptive behaviour. This often relies heavily upon the values of the doctor or the nurses involved. These values may be 'upper-middle-class' or 'institutional' in character. Behavioural assessment tries to be more objective, asking why the patient is unhappy with his behaviour or why it is upsetting to others. Where the patient does not recognise any problem, but others do, we must judge whether or not a real problem exists. This issue will be discussed more fully when we discuss ethics.

The information collected in this history tells the nurse *what* the problem is, in terms of behaviour, what other remedies have been tried, how big it is and what environmental factors are associated with its occurrence. The last section of the history explains why this is a problem for this patient.

The Problem Analysis

The next goal is to describe what happens when the patient engages in the behaviour. The nurse will try to identify what is happening around him, i.e. the events which precede and follow his behaviour.

Antecedents. The stimulus events which precede the behaviour are called antecedents. These can be sub-divided into the following categories:

(1) Physical: where the patient is just before the behaviour occurs.
(2) Social: what is happening around him. Does anyone say or do anything in particular? How many people are present? How are they interacting with the patient?
(3) Overt behaviour: what the patient is doing just before he begins engaging in the problem behaviour.
(4) Cognitive behaviour: what the patient is thinking just before performing the behaviour.
(5) Physiological: any special sensation felt by the patient, prior to the behaviour, e.g. sweating, muscle tension, etc.

Answers to these kinds of questions will indicate the 'setting' for the problem — what is happening outside and inside the person.

Consequences. The stimulus events which follow the behaviour are called consequences. These employ the same sub-headings as above:

(1) Where was the patient following performance of the behaviour?
(2) What did others do or say as a result of his behaviour?
(3) What did he do afterwards?
(4) What did he think about what had happened?
(5) How did he feel afterwards?

Functional analysis is rarely easy. People are inclined to say 'well nothing happened really . . . he just got up and hit me with the ash tray', or 'I was feeling OK one minute . . . and then all of a sudden I was gripped by this panic.' The same is true of consequential events. People may forget what happened afterwards, if it did not appear to be significant. The nurse is also faced with deciding how wide to extend the net of the analysis. The events or circumstances which are significantly related to the behaviour may be distanced in time and place. Mrs Smith might have had a row with her boss at work, been reprimanded and threatened with the sack. She may have thought about this incident all the way home and, *as she entered the house*, she may have started to become anxious. If we look too narrowly we may miss the significant antecedent and consequential events. Immediate events which occur with some regularity should be analysed first. If no obvious pattern emerges the 'net' should be widened gradually, until the significant events are isolated.

Redefinition of the Problem

The last task in the functional analysis is to redefine the problem using the information collected. The original 'fuzzy' description can now be translated into more objective terms. The 'panic attacks', 'psychotic outbursts', 'temper tantrums', etc., can now be described in terms of:

(1) what the patient says, does, thinks or feels;
(2) where he engages in this behaviour;
(3) who is present and what events are taking place;
(4) what usually happens before and . . .
(5) . . . what happens afterwards, which has a direct bearing on the behaviour;
(6) why this is seen as a problem.

This working definition summarises all the information from the functional analysis. Since the treatment will involve some kind of relearning, the assessment must spell out these situational 'variables' which will need to be taken into account in the design of the programme.

The Motivational Analysis

The nurse now proceeds to identify the patient's 'positive and negative reinforcers'. The nurse tries to identify the activities which the patient would most like to take part in, if he had a free choice. These are his 'positive reinforcers'. The other side of the reinforcement coin involves the activities which he would avoid, given a free choice. These are his 'negative reinforcers'. These can be divided into categories as shown on the schedule in Appendix 1. The first class concerns overt reinforcers, viz:

    consumable — food, drink, cigarettes, etc.

    tangible — records, possessions, toys, clothes, etc.

    persons — friends and enemies.

    places — cinema, park, swimming baths, etc.

    activity — games, concerts, doing homework, etc.

The nurse asks the patient, or other, to list 'likes' and 'dislikes' under the headings above. She can then draw up a list of most pleasing or displeasing activities or events. These potent reinforcers may play a large part in the eventual treatment programme.

In the second part of the analysis the nurse tries to define less obvious reinforcers. Although this analysis can be completed with the help of staff who know the patient well, there is a danger that they will provide only a list of 'opinions'. Ideally, this analysis should be completed with the help of the patient. Provided that the questions are phrased appropriately, there is no reason why some mentally handicapped people and longer-term psychiatric patients cannot participate in this analysis.

The nurse tries to define the patient's likes or dislikes, related to the six factors listed below. Although these are all constructs, they can be defined behaviourally, in terms of what the patient, or others, does, says, or thinks to himself.

(1) Independence. Does the patient enjoy independence, e.g. making decisions about when to get up, go to bed, what to wear, eat or do, etc. What sort of things does he say or think which indicates his like or dislike of independence.

(2) Peer approval. What does the patient like or dislike about his peer group, e.g. friends, workmates, fellow patients? What does he like or dislike them saying or doing? Do some of his peers give him special support or satisfaction? Does he enjoy being part of a group or gang, etc.

(3) Family approval. Does the patient enjoy the support and attention of his family, or not? Is there a special person in his family? What

does that person say or do which gives the patient a sense of satisfaction, pleasure or approval?

(4) Official approval. Does the patient enjoy, or dislike, the support or approval of people in authority, e.g. policemen, ward sister, headmaster, priest, etc.? What do these people do which gives satisfaction or causes annoyance?

(5) Success. Does the patient like to compete or win, e.g. is he competitive at work or play? Does he like to keep up with fashions etc? Does he enjoy feedback about how well he has done in exams etc? Does he dislike success? What does he say which suggests this?

(6) Personal appraisal. What does the patient like or dislike about himself? What is he proud or ashamed of? What would he like others to recognise, or to be unaware of, about himself?

The nurse should ask the patient, or other, to consider each heading in turn, giving some examples of the kind of reply she expects. Through discussion she should be able to define each factor in behavioural terms. For instance the patient might say 'I like to buy my own clothes . . . and decide where I want to go . . . and who goes with me. I like telling people what I think about things . . . even if they don't agree with me. I *hate* people telling me what to wear . . . and saying that I look silly. I don't like people telling me how I should behave either'. These sound like the sentiments of the typical teenager, but were taken from an interview with a 48-year-old mentally handicapped woman in hospital. These comments tell us a lot about the person behind the patient label. This information will be helpful in designing an appropriate treatment programme. In her case she would have to be given every opportunity to participate in her own programme. Indeed, from what she has said, the programme might fail completely if it was organised along traditional 'authority' lines.

This last part of the motivational analysis is not a personality test. We are not interested in the patient's personal constructs regarding 'independence', etc. We want to define more patterns of behaviour, whether shown by the patient or others. These positive or negative 'reinforcers' will be added to those listed in the first stage of the motivational analysis for possible use in the treatment programme.

Self-control Potential

In the next stage of the assessment, the nurse tries to find out if the patient has any behaviour which could be used to 'control' the problem. Where he has a chance to perform one behaviour — which could have pleasant *or* unpleasant consequences — but chooses to perform another,

he is demonstrating 'self-control'. Fighting can have pleasant consequences, e.g. when we punch an enemy on the nose. It can also have
unpleasant consequences, e.g. when we are fined for disturbing the
peace. A 'controlling' behaviour for fighting might be 'lighting up and
smoking a cigarette' or 'studying a newspaper'. These behaviours, which
are incompatible with fighting, are examples of *overt* self-control: they
can be observed by someone else.

The nurse is also interested in *covert* control. The simplest way to
find out if the patient uses such strategies is to ask him to list any
significant assets which he has acquired recently. These might be 'being
punctual, keeping fit, stopping smoking'. How did he gain these assets
and how does he maintain them? The patient might describe how he
stays away from other smokers, or walks in the opposite direction,
when he sees a tobacconist's. Can he increase his self-control by *thinking*?
The patient may use 'negatively reinforcing' thoughts like 'you want
a cigarette, but do you want lung cancer?' Or he may give himself
positive reinforcement by saying 'I've been really healthy recently . . .
I expect everyone is remarking on my strength of character in stopping
smoking'. This 'positive' thought may be used to stop him 'blotting his
copybook' at times of strong temptation.

An assessment of self-control potential usually can only be done
with the help of the patient. However, those close to the patient may
be able to show how he has controlled his behaviour in the past. This
information will be helpful in determining how much supervision the
patient will need during treatment and the extent to which he will be
able to participate.

Analysis of Social Relationships

The important people in the patient's environment are the 'significant
others'. The nurse needs to identify who they are and what their
relationship is with the patient, e.g. father, fellow patient, priest. This
list should include not only those who are in regular contact with the
patient, but also those, like distant relatives, whom the patient sees less
frequently. Such people may be able to reinforce some aspect of the
treatment, by sending a letter or telephoning the patient. The nurse
should note what this 'significant other' does *for* the patient: does he
provide support or is he a source of conflict? What sort of things does
this person do *with* the patient: do they go out together, play together,
argue with each other, or confide in each other?

Therapeutic Expectations

Finally, the nurse asks the patient, or significant other, what he expects from the therapy. What does he think the nurse is going to do for the patient? Such expectations are important. The nurse may have to point out unrealistic expectations, stating clearly, and sympathetically, why she cannot fulfil these for the patient. Alternatively, both nurse and patient may agree on the general aims of therapy, but may differ in terms of specific targets. Such a 'difference of opinion' should be acknowledged and an attempt made, through discussion, to agree on the goals of treatment. The patient may believe that he is going to receive some kind of 'talking cure', which will only require him to discuss his problems on a weekly basis. If the therapy is likely to involve him more than this, or in a wholly different way, this should be pointed out at the outset. Care staff, or parents, may think that the nurse is going to solve the patient's problems single-handed. If she hopes to enlist their support and assistance, then she must make this clear before proceeding further. In some cases the patient may be alarmed by the question. He may not be used to being asked what *he thinks* about his problem and may have no idea what is going to happen to him. Once again, the nurse must make it clear what the therapy will, or will not, involve.

The nurse should always allow some time at the end of the interview to summarise the information she has been given, if only to show that it has been heard and understood. The nature of this summary depends largely on the characteristics of the individual patient. However, the nurse should try to steer a course between being too technical and too condescending. Although it is no more than courtesy, it is worth emphasising the need to *thank the patient*, or other, for his help — and tolerance — during the interview.

The Assessment Summary

As soon as the functional assessment is complete the nurse should define the behaviours selected as targets for further assessment or eventual therapy. These would be listed along with details of the kind of *measures* which she considers would be most appropriate.

Target for assessment	*Measure*
'aggressive outbursts'	— frequency count, taken by ward staff on crisis incident record.

'social interaction'	— time-sample during free-time and mealtimes.
'assertive behaviour'	— Rathus assertiveness schedule given to patient.

The nurse should also specify the behaviour set as change-targets. These may be altered in future, depending on the outcome of the base-line. These are described in terms of their increase or decrease.

Target for change	*Method*
'decrease anxiety in crowds'	— stress inoculation training in clinic and exposure *in vivo*.
'increase appropriate spoon use'	— prompting, modelling and positive reinforcement.

These notes may be revised as further information is collected or as the programme is designed. However, they demonstrate that the nurse has gathered her thoughts about this patient and his problems, before proceeding to a new case or a new stage of the assessment. Appendix 1 shows a completed interview schedule, ending with a summary of the whole interview.

Summary of the Assessment Process

The assessment process described falls into three stages. In the initial interview the nurse gets to know something of the patient and his background and completes a simple 'thumbnail sketch' of his problems. Where the patient is unknown to the nurse this may take 30–40 minutes. If the nurse and patient are already acquainted, it may be much shorter. The global assessment provides some background details and may reveal 'new' problems. This assessment can be completed by care staff or next of kin, in the case of a 'dependent' patient. Where the patient completes it himself, it may take the form of a 'homework assignment'. The nurse's role here is to spend some time explaining the scales or questionnaires and analysing the information when they are returned to her.

The functional analysis looks more closely at the events which may be influencing the patient's behaviour. The second phase of this analysis is concerned with collecting information about the patient and his situation, which can be used in the design of the treatment programme.

Nurses often believe that they do not have the time to assess their patients, other than in the most cursory fashion. Where staff numbers are low this may well be true. However, in such situations an improved assessment method is not required, so much as a more realistic staffing policy. The assessment process described in this chapter can be modified to fit any nursing situation: hospital ward, community clinic or domiciliary visit. It serves as a framework for the analysis of almost any kind of problem, in any patient population. However, the repertoire is as yet incomplete. One important ingredient is missing: the skills and knowledge necessary to use the format efficiently and creatively. Any assessment is no more than a potential tool. It will provide a framework for the nurse to display her skills, but will rarely cover up her deficiencies.

Notes

1. Morganstern, R.D. 'Behavioural interviewing: the initial stages of assessment'. In: Hersen, M. and Bellack, A.S. (eds), *Behavioural Assessment* (Oxford, Pergamon Press, 1976).

2. Kanfer, F.H. and Saslow, G. 'Behavioural diagnosis'. In: Franks, C.M. (ed.), *Behaviour Therapy: Appraisal and Status* (New York, McGraw-Hill, 1969).

5 MEASUREMENT: FROM IDENTITY TO EVALUATION

> It is much to be regretted that habits of exact
> observation are not cultivated in our schools;
> to this deficiency may be traced much of the
> false reasoning and philosophy which prevails.
> — W. Humboldt

The *baseline* is the final part of the assessment process. Here we try to measure the problems which were defined in the functional analysis. The baseline is so called because it involves looking at the person's behaviour under natural conditions, before treatment begins. Knowing how much behaviour is shown under normal conditions gives us a base against which to evaluate the effects of treatment.

In the last chapter we discussed how the patient is assessed through interviewing or through the use of rating scales or questionaires. Although these methods give us an estimate — in the form of a general picture — they do not provide 'real' measures of the problem. They do not tell us how much behaviour is shown in different situations. Our estimate of the problem is turned into a real measure by recording the behaviour:

(1) where it normally occurs;
(2) at the time of day it normally occurs;
(3) under the conditions which normally prevail;
(4) using objective and reliable recording techniques.

In the baseline we measure the scale of the problem. If it is no more extreme than other people's behaviour, there may be no need for treatment. If the problem is sufficient to merit treatment the baseline will help us to judge whether or not the treatment works. In this sense, the baseline is the last stage of assessment and the beginning of the evaluation process.

Baseline

The Retrospective Baseline

Where the patient's behaviour is a threat to himself, or to those around him, a baseline should never be taken. Any self-injurious behaviour, such as head-banging or self-mutilation, should not be observed under baseline conditions. The same rule applies to the eating of rubbish or excreta or to any violent behaviour. Severely disturbed behaviour of this sort will be monitored by incident or accident records. By checking such records for details, dates and times, a baseline of sorts can be produced. Although these reports may not be as clear and objective as the observational methods we are about to discuss, they will provide a reasonable base against which to evaluate treatment. Where the patient is a danger to himself or others a retrospective baseline is more than adequate.

Preparing the Baseline

In the baseline we try to study the patient in his natural habitat, i.e. in the situations which give rise to his problem. We have stressed already the need to define the behaviour. It is important also that we define the *situation* in which it takes place. When people change from one situation to another, their behaviour also changes. Children who are 'holy terrors' at home may be 'little angels' at their grandparents' home. People who are anxious during an interview become calm and relaxed as they leave the building. Factors in the situation encourage certain behaviours to appear and discourage others. When the situation changes, we can expect the behaviour to change accordingly.

When preparing the baseline our first priority is to keep constant the conditions under which the behaviour is to be observed. Each observation should take place at the same time, in the same place, when similar activities are ongoing and when similar numbers of people are present. Of course it is impossible to keep all such conditions constant. However, changes should be kept to a minimum if marked changes in behaviour are to be avoided.

In some cases we may wish to measure how the patient behaves under different conditions. For instance, Mrs Smith complained of a 'fear of crowds'. Our baseline might measure how long she could stay in a crowded situation. However, we must first define 'a crowded situation': does that mean five, ten or one hundred people? By taking Mrs Smith to, for example, a shopping mall at different times of day on different days of the week, we could study her reaction to different sizes of crowd. Alternatively we could measure how 'fearful' she is in different situations, e.g. in the busy street as opposed to in a crowded shop.

A measure of Brian's incontinence would have to take account of several factors. It is not enough simply to record how often he wets himself. We must ensure that the conditions which may influence this behaviour are kept relatively constant. He may be incontinent more often when kept in the ward all day in comparison with the times he is outside playing. Alternatively, he may be incontinent more often when a lot of people are present, than when he is on his own. Our baseline would study his incontinence in a number of typical situations, in an attempt to isolate those which have a bearing upon the incontinence. In all these situations the amount of fluid taken each day would have to be strictly controlled, as this will influence his urinary output. A prescribed amount of fluid should be given in set amounts at specific times each day and a note regarding the need to control fluid intake should be attached to the observer's guidelines.

The Observer. We must also decide who will carry out the baseline. Will this be the patient himself, some relative or friend, or a nurse or nursing aide? The answer will determine the selection of the observational method and the kind of information which it will be possible to collect. If the patient observes his own behaviour he will be able to measure most of the behaviour patterns which an 'outsider' could study. He will also be able to monitor behaviour performed in private, as well as covert behaviour, such as thoughts and fantasies. Although the patient may be an excellent observer *in principle*, the format must be designed carefully. The measure should not be too complicated, should not take up too much of the patient's time and should not disrupt the natural 'flow' of the behaviour too much.

Where the baseline is completed by an 'outsider', more specific observations are possible. However, the expertise of the observer must be taken into account. If he or she has little experience of formal observation then the format may need to be as simple as that required for the patient himself. Where the observer is experienced, more complex forms of measurement are possible. In both cases the observational method should be 'cost-effective', providing a high return of information for a relatively small amount of effort. Where the observer is a nurse who normally works with the patient, extra care must be taken to ensure that the typical nurse-patient interaction pattern is not disrupted seriously. Any significant change in the nurse's behaviour will affect the patient also.

Guidelines. The observer must be given specific guidance about how to complete the observations; this applies to the patient as well as to a professional observer. These guidelines should be clear and brief, telling the observer where, when and how to take the measure. They should also make it clear what the observer should do with the information, once the record is complete.

Recording Equipment. Although sophisticated recording devices are available commercially to record complex patterns of behaviour or to 'translate', for example, muscle tension into sound frequencies, in general these are not used widely. The most practical observational methods are 'paper-and-pen' techniques. However, to use these methods well some basic equipment is essential.

(1) The record sheet: some kind of record format will be needed to make notes on the behaviour. This may be a standardised form, like the incontinence and self-feeding records shown in Figures 5.8 and 5.9. These may be used for a wide range of patients, who present with the same problem. In other cases, special record forms may need to be designed to suit the individual, e.g. where the patient is to be his own observer, or where a standardised record is inappropriate. Although record sheets are often A4 in size, small record cards — which the patient or staff member could carry in their pocket — may be more convenient. When selecting the recording format it is important to ask 'will this be *suitable* for recording the observations . . . and will it be *practical* in this situation?'

(2) The stopwatch: many digital wristwatches have in-built stopwatch facilities, which can be used to time the duration of behaviour precisely. Where careful measurement of minutes and seconds is not essential, an ordinary watch will be suitable. Where careful timing is required, a stopwatch is the most useful timepiece.

(3) The timer: a laboratory or kitchen timer is a helpful device for cueing the observer, when observations are arranged at regular intervals throughout the day. Whenever the timer rings, the observer collects the record form and begins the measure; on completion he re-sets the timer for the next observation. Again, many digital watches and calculators have this facility.

(4) The tally counter: a wide range of tally — or event — recorders are available for recording high-frequency behaviours. Where the

behaviour occurs repeatedly, in quick succession, making ticks on a piece of paper can be exhausting. The tally counter, which can be carried discreetly in the pocket, allows each occurrence to be registered without removing it. At the same time the person who is being observed need not be aware that the record is being taken.

(5) The tape recorder: an audio-cassette can be used to record the observer's 'commentary' on complex events, as they happen, and the tape can be analysed later, to extract specific measures. Where the patient is asked a series of questions, or is engaging in conversation, the tape recorder can be used to good effect. The recorder can also be used to cue observations, where a timer would be disruptive. A portable cassette recorder, worn over the shoulder, with an earpiece and a pre-recorded tape, can be used to instruct the inexperienced observer in what to look for and when to record, without alerting the patient.

(6) The clipboard: although this is not essential for all observations, it is invaluable for all A4-sized record sheets. In hospital settings, the clipboard can be hung in the duty station ready for the next observation. It is advisable to attach a pen or pencil to the board in case of emergencies.

Deciding What to Observe: The Crisis Incident Record

The functional analysis should tell us where, when and with whom the person usually engages in the behaviour. In some cases the behaviour may be shown across a wide range of situations and may appear unrelated to any particular events. In these cases some direct observation may be necessary before the baseline can be established. The crisis incident record (CIR) is used to analyse the situations under which the behaviour occurs. Figure 5.1 shows a typical record used by staff in a hospital and one for use by the patient himself.

The CIR is used each time the patient shows the target behaviour. This may be defined clearly, e.g. 'hitting other patients', or in more general terms, e.g. 'aggressive outbursts'. Each time the behaviour occurs the nurse notes briefly what the patient said and did, i.e. his behaviour. She also describes briefly the *antecedents* of the behaviour, i.e. what was happening before the behaviour occurred. She also notes the location, time of day and date. Finally she notes what happened *as a result* of the behaviour occurring, i.e. the *consequences*. If a note is made of the time the behaviour began and ended, the duration can be calculated. The second kind of CIR, used by the patient himself, includes what the patient was thinking and feeling, before and after the behaviour. If these records are completed over several days – or weeks,

Figure 5.1: Crisis Incident Report (CIR) — For Completion by Staff (A) and Patient (B)

(A) NAME .... WARD ....

DATE	ANTECEDENTS	BEHAVIOUR	TIME			CONSEQUENCES
			Started	Ended	Duration	
DATE	Where was the patient? What was happening around him?	What - exactly - did the patient do and say?				What happened as a direct result of his behaviour?

(B)

DAY & DATE	BEFORE	DURING	AFTER
	1. Where were you? 2. What was happening? 3. What were you doing? 4. What were you thinking? 5. How did you feel?	Describe what you actually did next	1. How did you feel? 2. What were you thinking? 3. Where were you? 4. What was happening?

depending on the frequency of the problem — some pattern of behaviour in relation to specific events may be isolated. When analysing the records, the nurse will be asking herself if the behaviour usually occurs in a certain place, at a certain time or after certain events have occurred. Answers to these questions will help structure the baseline observations. The record also gives valuable information about the effect of different consequences upon the behaviour: some appear to stop the behaviour; others may make it worse. In some cases the CIR is completed routinely after the functional analysis interview.

The CIR can also be used as a baseline measure. A frequency measure is possible if the record is completed *every time* the behaviour occurs. If the beginning and end of each behaviour are noted, then a duration measure can be produced. Where the same behaviour occurs across different situations (e.g. at home, in school or at play) the CIR may be the most practical form of baseline.

Direct Measurement

Frequency, Time and Severity

The main kinds of direct measures are *frequency*, which measures how often behaviour occurs, and *time*, which measures how long it lasts, or how long it takes to appear. A third measure, *severity*, is possible where the patient can measure his experience of the problem. Since this third measure is of more limited applicability, we shall discuss it first.

Rating the Problem

Where 'experience' is a significant aspect of the problem, as in feelings of anxiety or depression, the patient may describe this through the use of ratings. Since the rating relies on the patient's subjective experience the measures produced may be unreliable. However, if the patient's experience is significant, then his judgement of severity should be equally significant. Although ratings are not used exclusively with psychiatric patients like Mrs Smith, they are used most frequently with problems such as anxiety, obsessions and depression. However, many reports are now appearing describing their use with the mentally handicapped and more severely disturbed psychiatric patients.[1]

A rating scale can be produced to suit almost any problem. The patient is asked to record on the scale (e.g. 0–8) how he is feeling: e.g. anxious, angry or depressed. A description, at the lowest, highest and mid-point on the scale, helps the patient judge which point represents his feelings at present. For instance the scale might show 0 = 'relaxed, no anxiety' . . . 8 = 'extremely tense, anxiety unbearable'. The patient is then shown how to use the scale to monitor his experience of the problem, in different situations (see Figure 5.2).

Direct observation involves looking at the patient and making some kind of record of his behaviour. Although the methods described below are usually carried out by a trained person, there is no reason why they cannot be adapted to suit someone like Mrs Smith or Brian's mother. The first four methods require little practice to master them. The sampling methods have more specialised application and require more experience to use them effectively.

The Frequency Record. The frequency record — sometimes called event recording — involves counting the number of times the patient performs a behaviour, within a set period of time. We could record the number of times a person stands up, walks backwards and forwards or says 'Hello'. These would be recorded across an appropriate

Figure 5.2: Diary Sheet for Recording Anxiety in Everyday Situations

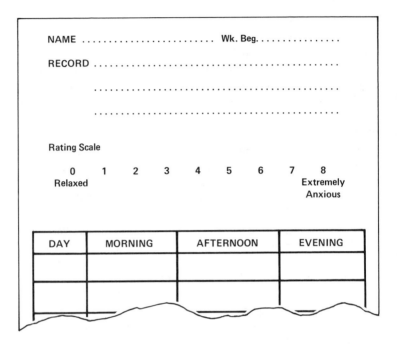

span of time. Where the patient can record covert behaviour he might count the number of times he had a certain class of thoughts. Mrs Smith might count her 'self-defeating' thoughts, using a tally counter in her pocket, e.g. 'I'll never be able to work again . . . (one) . . . I must get out of here right away . . . (two) . . . everyone is laughing at me . . . (three)' and so on. Brian's mother might record how often Brian sat down on the floor in shops, by making ticks on a card or at the top of her shopping list.

Although the frequency record is simple to use, the observer must know when the behaviour starts and stops, so that each individual occurrence can be counted. Some behaviours, like talking, sitting or writing, vary in length each time they occur and are not suitable for frequency recording. The frequency measure should only be used when the behaviour has an obvious start and finish and lasts for the same time each time it is shown. Behaviours like walking to the door, breaking a window, thumping the table and throwing a ball, all have a stable length and a clear beginning and end and are suitable for frequency recording.

Although the tally counter makes counting easier, there are other ways of recording frequency. A golf counter worn on the wrist, a knitting counter or shopping counter attached to the clipboard, or a card carried in the pocket, are other alternatives. A piece of tape applied to the back of the hand, to allow the recording of 'ticks', may be the simplest method. The type of recording should be selected to suit the situation. If the observer is free to study the patient for long periods, a record sheet divided into half-hourly intervals will show the distribution of behaviour across time. For instance, the behaviour might be shown repeatedly for a short period and may stop for several hours before another 'burst' of activity. If a simple record of frequency, per day or week, is all that is required, then a card or counter carried in the pocket will suffice.

The Latency Record.   In some cases it may be more important to record how long the person takes to begin or to finish the behaviour. One feature of 'depressed' or 'institutionalised' people is that they take a long time to answer questions. In such cases, a latency measure might be a useful measure of the problem. Handicapped children, learning to dress or to use cutlery, may also take a long time to perform such behaviours. In this situation the nurse might measure how long the child takes to finish dressing or eating, from the first instruction to do so, or from the moment he sat down at the table. The latency measure is very simple provided that the observer knows when to begin and end the timing. Discrepancies between different observers can be avoided by stating clearly when they should 'stop the clock', i.e. at the beginning *or* the end of the behaviour.

Duration Recording.   Where no obvious gap exists between separate occurrences, it is more appropriate to measure the time spent in the behaviour. If a person rarely speaks it is important to count how often he does say something. If he talks excessively it is more important to record how long he speaks for. Watching television, reading, pacing the floor and crying are all suitable for duration recording. A duration measure can also be used to clarify a frequency measure. For instance, a child might have four temper tantrums in one day. The duration record might show that these lasted for 8 minutes, 11 minutes, 14 minutes and 22 minutes respectively. The total time spent in temper tantrums adds another dimension to the measure of the problem. More significantly, the duration record reveals that they are getting longer each time.

A good working definition is essential for duration recording. The observer must know when the behaviour is present or absent. For instance, 'studying' could be defined loosely in terms of 'seated at desk with notebook and reading material'. Will this definition help the observer distinguish between studying and, for example, 'doodling and daydreaming'?

The Permanent Product Record.   The last of the simple methods is confined to those behaviours which leave behind a measurable product: words written, pieces of jig-saw fitted, pounds gained or lost, windows broken, etc. These can be measured *after* the person has completed the significant behaviour. This measure is valued by nurses who cannot spare the time to watch the patient engage in the behaviour. 'Smoking' can be measured by counting the number of butts left in an ashtray, 'dressing' by whether or not a child has tucked in his vest and shirt, and 'occupation' by the number of items assembled. However, the observer must devise some way of checking that the 'product' left is the result of the patient's behaviour and does not include the assistance or intervention of others.

In common with other measures the permanent product allows room for originality. A mentally handicapped child was referred for 'skin picking'.[2] The child repeatedly picked a large sore on his forehead, removing the dressing and healing tissue in the process. The wound bled for most of the day and the nurses said that they rarely caught him in the act of picking. Since it was not practical to observe him for long periods a permanent product measure was used. A small piece of sterilised paper tape was applied to the wound, overlapping it slightly. The tape simulated the scab necessary for healing and served as a measuring aid for 'picking'. The nurses applied the tape and checked the child a few minutes later. If it had been disturbed, one picking incident was recorded. The tape was re-applied and further checks repeated. For a mimimum of time and energy a representative measure of 'picking' frequency was possible.

Interval Recording.   Some behaviours are of short duration, occur often and vary in length. Eating, talking and playing can be as short as a few seconds or can last uninterrupted for many minutes. Since they vary in length a frequency count is impossible. Since they start, stop and start again, with only a brief pause, a duration measure would be too difficult. The alternative is to estimate the amount of time spent in the behaviour.

The procedure involves observing the patient for a set period (e.g. 20 minutes) which is broken down into small equal intervals (e.g. 10 or 20 seconds). The length of each interval should be short enough to ensure that only one occurrence of the behaviour is possible during the interval. Figure 5.3 shows a typical record sheet. The observer may record the behaviour *either* if it occurs at any time during the interval, or if it lasts for *most* of the interval.[3] At the end of the observation period the overall duration of the behaviour can be calculated as a percentage of the total intervals. The summary might show that the patient spent 32 per cent of the observation period talking to others. Since the behaviour may not have lasted for the full interal each time it occurred, it is not appropriate to translate this percentage into a 'length of time spent talking'.

Figure 5.3: Interval Record for Recording One Target Behaviour

NAME . . . . SITUATION . . . .

OBSERVER . . . . DATE . . . . FROM . . . . . TO . . .

TARGET BEHAVIOUR . . . .

INSTRUCTIONS

Observe patient for . . . . Record with a X if the target behaviour occurs during interval. Record with a O if behaviour does not occur. Record with slash marks (//) if patient absent.

1	2	3	4	5	6	7	8	9	10	11	12	13	14	15
16	17	18	19	20	21	22	23	24	25	26	27	28	29	30
31	32	33	34	35	36	37	38	39	40	41	42	43	44	45

109	110	111	112	113	114	115	116	117	118	119	120

SUMMARY % of intervals during which target occurred

Figure 5.4: Complex Interval Record

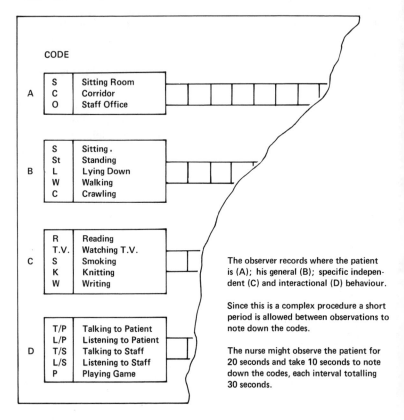

CODE

A
S	Sitting Room
C	Corridor
O	Staff Office

B
S	Sitting .
St	Standing
L	Lying Down
W	Walking
C	Crawling

C
R	Reading
T.V.	Watching T.V.
S	Smoking
K	Knitting
W	Writing

D
T/P	Talking to Patient
L/P	Listening to Patient
T/S	Talking to Staff
L/S	Listening to Staff
P	Playing Game

The observer records where the patient is (A); his general (B); specific independent (C) and interactional (D) behaviour.

Since this is a complex procedure a short period is allowed between observations to note down the codes.

The nurse might observe the patient for 20 seconds and take 10 seconds to note down the codes, each interval totalling 30 seconds.

Complex Interval Record. The interval record can also be used where different behaviours are grouped under an 'umbrella' title, such as 'social' or 'disruptive' behaviour. Figure 5.4 shows a typical format for monitoring social behaviour and the situation in which it occurs. To simplify the recording the behaviours have been categorised as follows:

(1) Mutually exclusive: those which cannot take place at the same time as another mutually exclusive behaviour. Standing and sitting are mutually exclusive; one cancels out the possibility of the other.

(2) Concomitant: other *independent* behaviours which can be performed together with mutually exclusive behaviour.

(3) Interactive: those which involve interaction with others.

Our example shows that in the first interval the patient was sitting, reading and listening to another patient in the television room. In the second interval he was still sitting, but was now talking to another patient and smoking. In the third interval he had left the chair and was standing by the window. This format would be used to measure the amount of observation time the patient spent in 'social' behaviour.[4]

The Time Sample. Where the behaviour lasts longer but is scattered across the day, a time-sample measure is more appropriate. Here the observer *visits* the situation at set intervals — e.g. every ten minutes or every hour — and records what the patient is doing at that time. The observer acts like a camera: she 'snaps' the action as soon as she arrives on the scene. The observer does not wait to see what the patient is going to do, but records what he is doing at that split second *at the end* of the observation interval.

Figure 5.5: Time-sample Record for Recording 'Engaged'/'Disengaged' Behaviour for Group of Individuals

INSTRUCTION: Observe each child every . . . . . minutes. Record child engaged (E) or disengaged (D).

Observe each child in order 1 - 10. If absent record with slash marks (//).

Child No.	1	2	3	4	5	6	7	8	9	10	11	12	13	14	15	E	D
1																	
2																	
3																	
4																	
5																	
6																	
7																	
8																	
9																	
10																	
11																	
12																	

Time – Sample No. / Percentage

Time-sampling is appropriate for behaviours lasting longer than five minutes, e.g. play, work and sleep. Where a number of behaviours are being measured the interval between each observation is adjusted to catch the shortest-lasting behaviour. If it is not possible to do this the time-sample is still feasible. However, the final measure will be only a rough estimate of the behaviour, since it may have occurred between the samples.

The time-sample can be adapted to study groups of people. Figure 5.5 shows a record for measuring 'engaged' and 'disengaged' behaviour. Engaged behaviour is defined as 'engaging in any appropriate action', e.g. playing, talking and laughing. Disengaged behaviour is defined as 'engaged in any inappropriate action', e.g. fighting, breaking toys or sleeping. Each patient is given a number on the record sheet (1 to 10). The observer visits the situation and records whether the first patient is engaged or disengaged. She then records each patient in turn, following the numerical order. The observer leaves and returns at the next 'sample' time. Each time she observes patient one first and patient number ten last. This ensures that the same length of time between 'samples' applies to each patient.[5]

The recording is analysed as a percentage of total observations. In our example one patient might be engaged 68 per cent of the time, whereas another might have been disengaged 90 per cent of the time, spending most of his time fighting or sleeping. The time-sample is often paired with the permanent product measure, e.g. hourly or half-hourly checks on incontinence and hourly checks on work output.

Checklists.   One of the simplest observational methods is the checklist. This is used to measure either/or situations: has the patient made his bed? (or not); are his buttons fastened?; has he combed his hair? This record, usually aimed at everyday living skills, assesses whether or not the patient's behaviour is 'appropriate' (see Figure 5.6). Although very simple to complete, the checklist can be wasted if observers do not agree on the definition of 'appropriate'. A sample list of 'appropriate' and 'inappropriate' examples for each behaviour on the checklist should be given to each nurse to ensure agreement between different observers.

The Selection of Methods.   The selection of the most appropriate measure is determined by: the nature of the problem; the situation in which it occurs; the person acting as observer; and the time available. As we have shown, some behaviours can be counted whereas others need to be timed. Sampling methods are used where the behaviour is

Figure 5.6: Simple Checklist of Measure-selected Everyday Living Skills

NAME . . . .   WARD . . . .

Record X if satisfactory; O if unsatisfactory

A : HYGIENE

	1	2	3	4	5	6	7	8	9	10	11	12
Face Clean												
Hands Clean												
Teeth Brushed												

B : APPEARANCE

	1	2	3	4	5	6	7	8	9	10	11	12
Hair Combed												
Clothes Clean												
Buttons Fastened												
Shoes Tied												

variable in length and irregular in frequency or where observer time is limited.

In general, where frequency or duration measures are taken, only one or two behaviours can be measured in the single patient. Although they are simple to use, they may not be 'cost-effective'. Although sampling methods require more skill in preparation and practice in their administration, they may be more economical for nurses concerned with groups of patients. In certain cases the nurse may be able to enlist the support of the patient and his 'significant others' in completing observations. The patient might measure one aspect of the problem, his family and friends another, and the nurse a third aspect. The final measure would be drawn from an evaluation of the different measures.

Observational Packages

Our case studies involve a range of problems of living, each needing a different kind of measure. In some cases this could be taken by the patient, over a few days. In other cases, the behaviour may need to be studied over several weeks, by staff specially trained in the analysis of behaviour. To compare the use of different methods we shall look briefly at some of the problems presented by our patients.

The Measurement of Anxiety.   Mrs Smith's initial assessment showed that she felt anxious in a number of situations. The nurse would now ask her to help her collect more information about the problem, to help evaluate the treatment programme. When a patient is asked to fill in forms or participate in measuring his own behaviour, he may feel a little anxious, whether or not this is his presenting problem. In order to allay such natural fears the nurse must give clear and concise instructions as to what is required of the patient. These instructions should be free of jargon, in language he can understand. A few minutes spent discussing with Mrs Smith what *she* means by anxiety, will ensure that both are speaking the same language and that the patient is in no doubt as to what she is being asked to monitor.

The simple diary format, shown in Figure 5.2, might be the best system to use in this case. Mrs Smith could note what she has been doing each day and how she felt in each situation. Since part of her problem is the avoidance, or poor tolerance, of stressful situations, it may be worth measuring how long she can stay in such situations. If progress is likely to be slow at first, the nurse might ask Mrs Smith to time herself as accurately as possible, so that even slight changes for the better can be evaluated. These times can be noted on the diary sheet beside the anxiety ratings. Mrs Smith also described her 'negative-thinking' strategies. The nurse must decide whether or not she should record these at this stage; If a record of these thoughts is considered worthwhile, they could be counted using a tally counter. If Mrs Smith used the CIR (Figure 5.1b) to record her daily activities, she could add 'what I am thinking' to the record of her anxiety rating.

Since Mrs Smith's problem has been static for some time the baseline may take only a few days to complete. At the end of this time the nurse will know how anxious she is at different points on her hierarchy, how long she can tolerate such situations and what she is thinking before, during and after exposure to stress.

The Measurement of 'Unassertiveness'.   Mrs Smith also complained of difficulties in her personal relationships. This had been the root of her troubled marriage and is now evident in her strained relationship with her mother. She feels that she gets 'trodden upon' in any disagreement with her mother and cannot cope with her bossy attitude. Since she could not tell her this directly, she took an overdose in an attempt to show her how unhappy she was. The Rathus assertiveness schedule confirms that she has difficulties in conflict situations. If this was reapplied later in the treatment it could be used as an evaluation measure. However, the nurse might want to know more about these coping difficulties. What does the patient do which shows that she is 'unassertive'? In order to assess this more precisely the nurse might arrange a role-play of a typical conflict situation, asking another nurse – of about the same age as the patient's mother – to act out the scene with her. The patient's verbal and non-verbal 'assertiveness' could then be rated: does she give appropriate eye-contact, show appropriate facial expression, speak loud enough or clear enough, stand appropriately?[6] This assessment will identify the skills which need specific coaching. To complete the picture, Mrs Smith might be asked to record how often 'conflicts' occurred at home, rating how well she handled the situation. Although a separate record card could be used, this information could be included on the CIR.

The Measurement of Social Excesses.   Sally showed a combination of deficits and excesses of behaviour. She spends a lot of time asking staff and other patients for cigarettes and much of her day asleep in the dayroom. 'Begging for cigarettes' could be measured by a simple fre-quency record. A nurse could be allocated to observe Sally, recording each occurrence of the behaviour. Alternatively, each nurse could note down each time Sally asked her, or a patient within earshot, for a cigarette. Although there is a chance that the same incident could be recorded by separate observers, this may be a more accurate record since it covers a wider area of the ward.

'Begging' could be measured as a daily total: staff leaving their record cards, when they go off duty, to be totalled by the nurse in charge of Sally's care. However, since she also spends a lot of time asleep, it might be interesting to see how her 'begging' varies throughout the day. The frequency could be tallied for each hour and recorded on an hour-by-hour chart. This would still provide a daily total, but would also indicate peak times when the behaviour is more prevalent. These times would become the focus for the treatment programme. Since Sally's 'begging' waxes and wanes, according to the availability of cigarettes, it would be advisable to run the baseline for at least two weeks or until a pattern established itself on the hourly chart.

The Measurement of Social Deficits.   Sally is also loathe to spend time with other patients or in ward activities. Since the nurses can predict when this behaviour will be shown, either a time-sampling or interval recording format would be appropriate. Nurses might measure whether Sally spends her time 'actively' or 'passively' using the engaged-disengaged format shown earlier. If they wished to study her avoidance of social situations more closely, an interval record might be more appropriate. Thirty minutes could be spent watching what Sally does when staff and other patients try to engage her in conversation. A record sheet listing the kind of social behaviours shown in Figure 5.4 could include the avoidance strategies which Sally usually reserves for such situations.

Since Sally's 'apathy' extends throughout the day it might be worth measuring her performance of other routine activities, e.g. self-care and domestic routines. Portues[7] has produced a recording format which the patient (in this case called Pat) carries in her handbag; this is checked and scored by staff at different times and locations throughout the day (see Figure 5.7). Although the patient is not monitoring her own behaviour she is given the responsibility of carrying the record sheet. She is also acutely aware that the staff are recording her behaviour. The design of this recording format takes into account a range of target behaviours and the patient's ability to understand and participate, to a limited extent, in the assessment.

Although Sally might be able to participate to a very limited extent in the baseline measure, for others like Brian, this will not be possible. In his case all measures will need to be taken by care staff or his parents. One of his major problems is his 'hyperactivity'; this disrupts his engagement in play, as well as routines like eating and dressing. Since he will not stay long in one place, it may be worth measuring how long he will *sit* on the toilet, at the table or on the floor, when asked to do so. Since most of his training needs will depend upon simple instruction-following and staying in one place long enough to learn something, a duration measure of sitting should prove helpful.

Brian's limited feeding skills could be measured using the kind of direct-observation rating scale shown in Figure 5.8. Since his eating skills are not likely to vary from one day to the next, two or three ratings of breakfast, dinner and tea, will give an overall eating skill score and will identify his major difficulties.

Incontinence would also be a major headache for both staff and parents. A first requirement in the assessment would be to exclude any physical reason for the problem, by arranging a medical examination. In the baseline the nurse would want to measure the number of times

Figure 5.7: A Personalised Token System

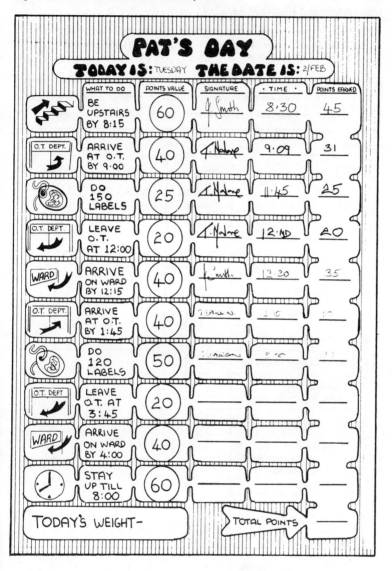

Figure 5.8: Example of Spoon-feeding Checklist Using Direct Observation and Rating Scale

INSTRUCTIONS : Score each stage (A — N) upon ASSISTANCE required to complete.

SCALE
0 — Refuses to Perform 3 — Requires Gestural Prompt
1 — Requires Full Physical Prompt 4 — Requires Verbal Prompt
2 — Requires Partial Physical Prompt 5 — Performs Unaided

NAME . . . .

WARD . . . . . .

		Date. . . . . Course No. 1	2	3	Date. . . . . Course No. 1	2	3	Date. . . . . Course 1	2
A	Walks to Table								
B	Sits at Table								
C	Picks up Spoon								
D	Fills from Plate								
E	Lifts to Mouth								
F	Removes from Mouth								
G	Leaves on Plate								
H	Picks up Bread (etc.)								
I	Takes Bites								
J	Removes from Mouth between Bites								
K	Raises Cup to Mouth								
L	Drinks 'Mouthfuls'								
M	Replaces between Drinks								
N	Leaves Table								
	Total Score (A — N)								

Figure 5.9: Incontinence Record Chart

NAME . . . . WARD . . . . . . Wk. Beg. . . . .

INSTRUCTIONS:

1. Give patient . . . . . .mls fluid at times marked with *

2. Each ½ hour check patient and record code viz : (In Column A)

   W : Wet   W/S : Wet & Soiled
   S : Soiled   D   : Dry

3. At toilet times (marked with ▲) record viz : (In Column B)

   U : Urinated   U/D : Urinated & defaecated
   D : Defaecated   N   : Did nothing

		MON		TUES		WED		THUR		FRI		SAT		SUN	
		A	B	A	B	A	B	A	B	A	B	A	B	A	B
	7.30														
*	8.00														
▲	8.30														
	9.00														
	9.30														
	10.00														
*	10.30														
▲	11.00														
	11.30														
	12.00														
*	12.30														
▲	1.00														
	1.30														
	2.00														

Brian was incontinent each day and where and when these incidents occurred. These 'peak-times' will help establish the best times to operate the programme. Since he is unlikely to be incontinent more than once an hour, hourly checks – recording 'dry' or 'wet' – would be adequate. However half-hourly or quarter-hourly checks would identify the time of urination more precisely (see Figure 5.9). Where it is available a portable urine-alarm[8] would signal each incontinent episode as it occurred. As we have noted already, it is important to control fluid intake, so that 'output' does not vary too much from one day to the next. If Brian has no control over his bladder, it will empty once a certain threshold is reached, at a certain time after fluid intake. If fluid intake is monitored carefully and hourly time-sampling checks are instituted, the nurse will be able to establish the 'peak-times' along with an overall frequency of incontinence. The whole process will require an investment of only two or three minutes each hour.

The Validity and Reliability of Observations

The examples above illustrate a major problem in assessment: how do we know that we have measured what we wanted to measure? Most of the problems referred to involve *constructs* rather than specific behaviours, e.g. apathy, anxiety, hyperactivity and unassertiveness. When planning baseline observations we must ask ourselves, for example, 'Is the length of time Brian spends sitting each day representative of his hyperactivity?'

In Sally's case the staff identified a single problem at the outset: begging for cigarettes. However they also described her as 'disruptive'. This construct could cover socially embarrassing behaviour such as 'begging for cigarettes'. Are the nurses concerned only with the begging problem? If not, it may be more appropriate to measure all socially embarrassing behaviour.

Mrs Smith might say that her 'coping' difficulties involve not knowing what to say in an argument. Does this mean that 'assertiveness' involves only verbal behaviour? Observation of the patient in a role-play might show deficiencies in non-verbal communication – e.g. eye-contact, gestures, facial expression – which would have to be taken into account in measuring assertiveness.

If the observer does not measure *significant* behaviour, then the real problem is not being studied. Similarly, if the measures taken are inaccurate, then the extent of the problem is still unclear and evaluation of the treatment will be impossible. Where the patient is his own observer we must trust him to complete the measures conscientiously.[9] Where observations are taken by staff in hospital *reliability checks*, or probes, should be arranged at intervals throughout the baseline. The nurse's observations may be inaccurate for a number of reasons:

(1) The behaviour may be poorly defined: one nurse may be recording one behaviour, while another is recording a slight variation of this.

(2) The recording format may be confusing or over-complicated; this may lead to errors, or may overwhelm the nurse completely.

(3) The nurse may have been given inadequate instruction in the use of the format.

(4) If the observations have been running for some time without review sessions, some observers may have changed the format slightly to suit themselves.

(5) The observations may be wholly accurate, but may have been analysed incorrectly.[10]

Observer Effect.   The mere presence of an observer can change the patient's behaviour. If we see someone filming us in the street, we may walk more erect or adjust our hair. During the early stages of baseline the same disruption can take place, the patient changing his behaviour as soon as he sees the observer. This effect will fade through time as the observer becomes just another aspect of the environment. Unnecessary observer effect can be prevented by making the observations as discreet as possible. However, in any situation, early recordings should be consigned to the waste-basket, using these sessions as mere 'dummy runs'.

Summary

The baseline involves taking a measure of the problem, in the patient's natural surroundings and in the situations where the problem usually shows itself. This measure may be taken by the patient, by those caring for him, or by those currently living with him. In each case the observer will want to use the simplest recording method, one which will provide the information required, for the minimum of effort. Although very simple measures exist, in some cases more complex measures may be more 'cost-effective', especially where complex patterns of behaviour or groups of patients are concerned.

Where the patient is observing himself, an everyday 'diary' or note-book format can be adapted to record the significant details of everyday experience, related to the problem. Ratings of severity, success or general competence, can be added to these diary-notes. Where trained staff are involved in hospital treatment the record format may resemble more traditional clinical measures, checklists and charts being used to record behaviour economically through ticks or scores on a record sheet. In either situation the aim of the baseline is to measure the rela-tive severity, frequency or length of the behaviour.

In most cases single observations of individual behaviours would reveal very little. Due to the complexity of most patients' problems, a package of observational measures is often indicated. In some cases standardised measurement systems may be applied to commonly occur-ring problems. In other cases, a special format may need to be designed to suit the patient and his situation. In every case the nurse must pay close attention to the validity and reliability of the measures produced. Has she measured the 'problem' which she first set out to measure? Are her observations an accurate representation of the problem?

Notes

1. Standardised rating scales are used increasingly in the preliminary stages of assessment for social skills training. See: Eisler, R.M., Blanchard, E.B. and Williams, J.G. 'Social skills training with and without modelling for schizophrenic and non-psychotic hospitalized psychiatric patients', *Behaviour Modification*, vol. 2, no. 2 (April 1978), pp. 147–72.

2. Barker, P. and Hunter, M.H. 'Minor self-mutilation', *Nursing Times* (7 April 1977), pp. 500–2.

3. If the interval is adjusted to suit the average duration of the behaviour, it should occupy the *majority* of that time interval. If the behaviour occurs only briefly during the interval, this suggests that the interval is too long and the resulting measure may be inaccurate.

4. 'Apathy' in hospitalised schizophrenics was originally defined and measured by use of a similar time sampling method. See: Schaeffer, H.H. and Martin, P.L. 'Behavioural therapy for "apathy" of hospitalized schizophrenics', *Psychological Reports*, vol. 19 (1966), pp. 1147–58.

5. The sequential time sample method described was used to study the social behaviour of hospitalised children, across a range of situations. See: Barker, P., Docherty, P. and Hird, J. ' "Showing an improvement": an examination of variables central to the token economy system', *International Journal of Nursing Studies*, vol. 17 (1980), pp. 25–37.

6. A helpful observational rating scale for use by nursing staff in social skills training is given in Liberman, R.P., King, L.W., De Risi, W.J. and McCann, M. *Personal Effectiveness: Guiding People to Assert Themselves and Improve their Social Skills* (Champaign, Illinois, Research Press, 1975).

7. Portues, C. 'The use of self-monitoring with a hospitalised psychotic patient', *CCNS Course Reports* (unpublished report, Royal Dundee Liff Hospital, 1981).

8. For a description of use, see: Foxx, R.M. and Azrin, N.H. *Toilet Training the Retarded* (Champaign, Illinois, Research Press, 1973).

9. Research has shown that the mere act of studying one's own behaviour closely causes it to change. For a review of 'reactivity' see: Kazdin, A.E. 'Reactivity of self-monitoring. The effect of response desirability, goal setting and feedback', *Journal of Consulting and Clinical Psychology*, vol. 42, no. 5 (1974), pp. 704–16.

10. For further reading on the reliability of direct observation see: Costello, A.J. 'The reliability of direct observation', *Bulletin of the British Psychological Society*, vol. 26 (1973), pp. 105–8.

6 DESIGNING THE TREATMENT PROGRAMME

Either I will find a way, or I will make one.
– Sir Philip Sidney

Planning the Intervention

Once the baseline is complete the nurse can begin planning the intervention. She has reached the end of the assessment which began at the initial interview (see Figure 6.1). The problem was described first, only in fuzzy terms. Secondly, at the end of the functional assessment it was broken down into its component parts: each of these was labelled with a 'working definition'. Thirdly, in the baseline the behaviours were measured and a clear picture of the problem emerged. All three phases will be used in the design of the treatment programme. To help streamline the design stage the nurse will ask the following questions:

(1) What is the nature of the problem?
(2) What should be the final treatment goals?
(3) When can treatment begin?
(4) How should the programme be organised?
(5) Which change-techniques would be appropriate?
(6) How should the programme be evaluated?
(7) Will the programme raise any ethical implications?

No treatment programme can proceed without answering these questions. In some cases they will be answered quickly. Where the programme involves only the nurse and the patient, an hour's discussion – at home, on the ward or at a clinic – may suffice. In other settings detailed treatment proposals may be needed for discussion at a multi-disciplinary case conference. Where children are concerned, the approval and co-operation of the parents may be required. Although hospital-based programmes may require greater planning, neither proposals nor discussions need be lengthy. Indeed, since the main aim is to offer the patient help, there is every reason to keep these brief. Careful answering of the seven questions above should help streamline any discussion, by addressing the key issues at the outset.

Figure 6.1: Clarification of the Problem

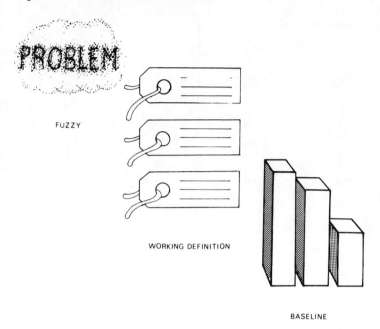

FUZZY

WORKING DEFINITION

BASELINE

Translating the Baseline

The information collected during construction of the baseline represents a picture of the patient's problem. Before designing the treatment programme the nurse must summarise this information. The simplest way to do this is in the form of a line graph (see Figure 6.2). This will show the relationship between *time*, shown along the horizontal axis, and the *measure*, shown on the vertical axis. The graph illustrates how the behaviour increases, or decreases, across the days or weeks of the observation period.

The average measure, or *mean*, can be calculated by dividing the total by the number of observations. Since the nurse does not know how high the behaviour will rise or how low it might fall, the graph should not be prepared until the observations are completed. If data are graphed as the baseline progresses the scale may turn out to be too long or too short. This is illustrated in Figure 6.3. Although the measures are identical, the problem appears to be more severe in one graph than in the other. In general, the scale should extend only a few

Figure 6.2: Converting Numerical Data into Graph Form

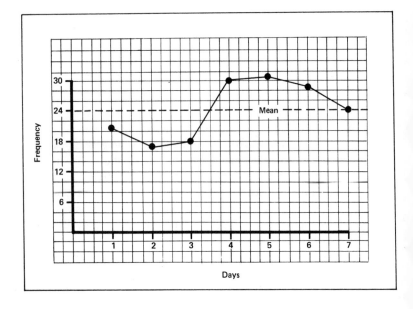

OBSERVATION DATA

Day No.	Frequency of Behaviour
1	20
2	17
3	18
4	30
5	31
6	28
7	24
Total	168

$$\text{Mean} = \frac{168}{7} = 24$$

Figure 6.3: Selecting an Appropriate Scale to Illustrate the 'Trend' of Observation Data

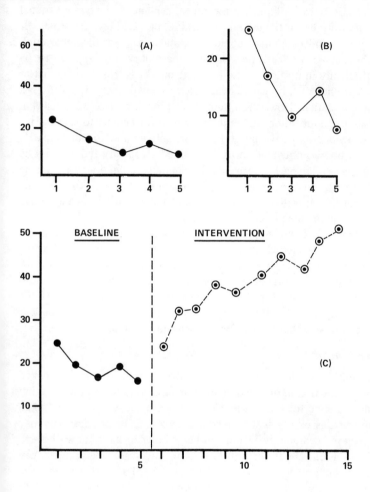

points beyond the highest measure; in this case the scale need not extend beyond 35. If the behaviour is expected to *rise* during treatment, a longer scale would be used to take this into account (see Figure 6.3C).

The Nature of the Problem

So far we have discussed the patient's problems in terms of excesses or deficits of behaviour. The patient either *does not* show behaviour which is desirable or in some way to his advantage, or he shows behaviour which is inappropriate or to his disadvantage. Although few problems are clearly a case of one or the other, genuine skill or motivational deficits can be distinguished by asking the acid-test question: 'If his life depended upon it, could the patient perform the behaviour?' If the answer is 'Yes' then he has the ability, but appears to be insufficiently motivated to use it. If the answer is 'No' then no matter how hard he tried, he would be unable to show the behaviour. This is a clear skill deficit. However, a number of problems involve limited skill *and* limited motivation. A 'mute' patient might be able to speak if his life depended on it. He might, however, only be able to call 'help'. He may be poorly motivated to use his limited vocabulary and may not be keen on developing his verbal skills. Similarly, a child may be unable to tie his shoe-laces. Although the problem involves a lack of skill, he may not be motivated to acquire the skill and may need some incentive for learning to take place.

Figure 6.4 shows the kind of questions which the nurse can use to isolate the obstacles which may be preventing the patient from showing the target behaviour. In some cases the obstacle will be lack of knowledge or ability. In others, it will be a lack of motivation. In other cases the patient may be obstructed by circumstances; he may not have the opportunity to show the behaviour. In some other cases the patient may be unaware that others view his behaviour as a 'problem'.

The Nature of Anxiety

Mrs Smith's problems were first described as skill deficits. She talked about how she *couldn't* go shopping or face up to her mother or think about planning for the future. However, since she was once able to go shopping this clearly is a motivational problem. By contrast, she may never have been able to face up to her mother or have known how to make decisions about her future. In both these cases the problem may derive, wholly or in part, from a lack of skill. Mrs Smith says that she feels anxious whenever she goes shopping, is involved in a conflict with her mother or contemplates her future. The nurse must question the role played by anxiety in each of the three areas. In the first, anxiety may be obstructing her from doing things she was once capable of doing and which she is wholly competent to perform. Where her mother is concerned she may have tried to 'stand up for herself', but found her performance lacking in some respect. When faced with repeated conflicts, her anxiety increases, since she is acutely aware of her limitations in handling the situation. In the third area she may feel

Figure 6.4: Skill and Motivational Deficits

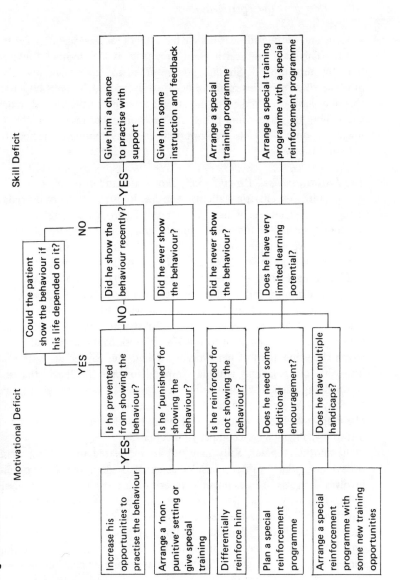

anxious and depressed because she has rarely practised planning for the future. This task was carried out originally by her mother followed later by her husband. She has now returned to dependence upon her mother. When she tries to make her own decisions, she feels hopeless: this may have been linked to her suicide attempt. In this case although she is able to make some plans and decisions, she may be unable to make the ones she feels are important and may require some specific help in this area.

The Institutionalised Patient.   Sally shows the kind of problems typical of long-term psychiatric patients. She has lost many of her everyday living skills. These may have been eroded through a long stay in a 'custodial' setting or may be a spin-off from other 'problems of living'. She may have lost the ability to cook, wash her own clothes, carry on a conversation or plan ahead and solve everyday problems. The ward staff may have tried to give Sally, and other patients, more responsibility for planning and conducting their own lives. However, Sally, like many others, may be unable to pick up where she left off so many years ago. Although she is no longer obstructed by an institutional system, she may need time to practise these skills under careful supervision. In some areas of her everyday living, she may be unaware that her behaviour is lacking and may respond to some 'feedback' that she is not doing particular behaviours often enough or well enough. In view of Sally's diagnosis, the kind of instruction or help with forward-planning, which she requires, will need to take careful heed of her memory span and any accompanying deficits.

In another respect, Sally may not be motivated to perform these behaviours, which others consider essential or desirable. Her routine involves doing as little as possible, meeting her own criteria of 'survival' skills. This may look like 'apathy' to us, but may be simple 'cost-effectiveness' as far as the patient is concerned. At other times she may show 'maladaptive' behaviour, like repeatedly asking for cigarettes. These behaviours may be the simplest ways she knows of getting something which she wants. Since more appropriate behaviour is likely to require more effort on her part, Sally may need to be motivated actively, perhaps by controlling the availability of the things which she likes. Since she is being asked to make a special effort Sally will, like most of us, expect us to 'make it worth her while'.

The Dependent Relationship.   Although Brian is still young, his problems may appear intractable, since he has probably behaved this way all his life. It is more than likely that he has never shown any of the target behaviours, which we would list as desirable. For instance, he has not mastered the intricacies of knife and fork use and rarely eats without making a mess. In addition to formal training, Brian will need more opportunities to practise these skills. Both staff and parents must change their orientation from 'caring for a dependent child' to 'training for independence'.

Staff also comment that he 'can't sit still for a minute'. Do they mean this literally? Could he sit still if his life depended upon it? Perhaps he will sit still if given something which interests him, if only for a minute or two. If we assume that Britain has acquired the skill of, for example, sitting on request, we must now identify the kinds of things — such as food, toys or activities — which will motivate him to do this for longer periods of time and more often.

The information which has been collected on Brian's incontinence requires a similar analysis. Is he incontinent each day? Is this always at the same times? Are there occasions when he appears to control his bladder? If his fluid intake is controlled, some pattern of incontinence should emerge. However, if the frequency varies from day to day — or if he passes small amounts of urine in quick succession — Brian may be controlling the extent of his incontinent behaviour. Perhaps the attention given by staff when changing and showering him after an incontinent episode, has some effect on the pattern of the behaviour. If so, this attention may need to be reallocated to motivate him to become continent. Even if this were so, Brian may still lack the ability to perform the many complex actions required in making use of the toilet. In this case continence training would involve both skill and motivational factors.

In this first stage of planning the nurse is asking herself about the kinf of *help* the patient will need to achieve the goals which have been set. Will he need to learn new skills, practise old ones, or increase the frequency of 'dormant' behaviours, which are conspicuous by their absence?

The Treatment Goals

During compilation of the baseline, problems were measured to help set more specific goals and to evaluate the treatment programme. The initial assessment may reveal that the patient lacks certain skills or is not motivated to show established patterns of behaviour. In judging what the baseline says about the problem the nurse must select realistic targets for the patient. She must consider not only the level of behaviour at present, but also how long it has been a problem of this stature. If the patient has only recently become troubled by anxiety there is a good chance that it can be brought easily within 'normal limits', no matter how severe it is at present. If the problem is long-standing and has proved resistant to other forms of treatment, a more realistic goal might be to try to reduce the problem, rather than to eliminate it altogether.

Where problems are complicated by association with some organic pathology, as in Sally's case, the nurse must question seriously the realistic goals for this patient. Treatment goals might be equally conservative in Brian's case. His lack of everyday living skills may be linked to attention deficits or distractibility, both of which may be greater handicaps than intellectual deficit. Sitting could be encouraged, not as an end in itself, but to provide a basis upon which to build other skills requiring command-following and attentional control.

Realistic treatment goals must take into account the resources available, as well as the nature of the problem. Many authors have described near-miracle cures with profoundly disturbed children.[1] However such successes are rarely achieved in the typical health service ward. In the understaffed and overcrowded hospital setting, there is a definite ceiling on the bounds of possibility. Although this warning should not be ignored, it should not be seen as an excuse to be defeatist. However, the need for realistic goal setting cannot be over-emphasised. The moral is to aim for goals which can be achieved with some degree of certainty. The result will cheer both nurse and patient and will fuel efforts to make further small gains.

Ending Baseline and Beginning Treatment

As we noted in the last chapter the baseline can, in some cases, act like a form of treatment. The simple act of observing oneself or being observed can produce a change in behaviour. For some people this change may become permanent. We have all heard people say 'I can keep my weight steady providing that I watch what I eat'. The same principle may be used by people who tend to drink, smoke or gamble too much. They can keep their excess behaviour within limits by monitoring it. When people are being watched closely the effect on their behaviour may be more dramatic. The observed person reacts to the presence of the observer by behaving differently. He may continue showing the target behaviour, at a higher or lower level than he would normally, or may change to a completely different pattern of behaviour. This 'reactivity' to observation — whether from the inside or

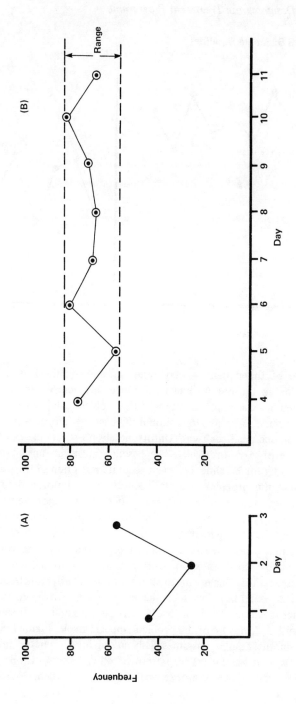

Figure 6.5: Frequency of 'Cigarette-begging' per day

Figure 6.6: Stable Baselines

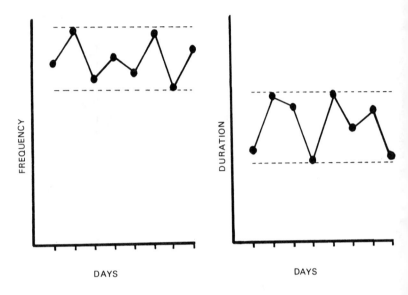

outside of the patient — may wear off quickly, the behaviour soon returning to the pre-baseline level. Once this observer effect has disappeared more accurate measures of the problem will be possible.

Most nurses ask 'how long should the baseline run for — two or three days, or one week or two?' Unfortunately no strict rule can be made in terms of days or weeks. The baseline must run until the picture provided by the baseline data is an accurate reflection of the problem.

Where the problem is a skill deficit, there is no need to observe the patient more than two or three times. If he cannot use a knife and fork correctly, his performance will be much the same each mealtime. Providing that the patient's behaviour is similar on each observation, the training phase may begin immediately. Where the behaviour varies from one day to the next, or from one situation to another, the nurse must assume that this is a motivational problem. Different circumstances appear to determine whether the behaviour is performed or not, or whether it is done 'well' or 'badly'. In this situation the baseline must run until the measure of the problem appears stable. Figure 6.5 shows a graph of the number of times Sally asked for a cigarette on the first three days of baseline. The pattern of 43, 27 and 49 is not stable; it is quite erratic. Over the next week (graph B) the behaviour does not

Figure 6.7: Ascending and Descending Baselines

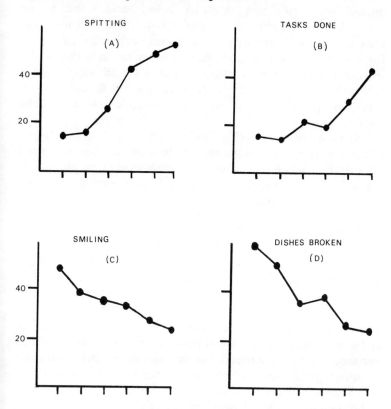

level out, but a definite pattern emerges. The range of 'begging' is between 59 and 80 per day. The lower frequencies shown over the first three days could well be an illustration of observer effect. Since these low frequencies are not registered again, the moral of the story is obvious. If only three days measures had been taken the average frequency of 'begging' would have been only 40. When the baseline runs until some stability is shown, the average becomes much higher – at around 70. Since the main aim of the baseline is to judge the *real size* of the problem, we must take care to avoid any false picture.

Figure 6.6 shows examples of stable baselines. Although the frequency and duration measures are not the same each day, they show a stable pattern, never rising or falling below certain levels.

Ascending and Descending Baselines.   In some cases measures may increase slowly across each observation, as in Figure 6.7. Since the aim is to reduce the frequency of 'spitting', the nurse does not have to wait until the behaviour stabilises. The treatment could begin on day six. However if the goal was to increase the behaviour, as in Figure 6.7b, she would have to wait for stability or until the behaviour began to descend in frequency. In the graph the child is steadily increasing the number of tasks he does each day without any specific treatment being applied.

The same rule applies when baselines are descending, as in Figure 6.7c and d. In Figure 6.7c the aim is to increase the behaviour; since it is currently descending, treatment can begin at any time. However in Figure 6.7d the maladaptive behaviour is dropping naturally; this rules out the need for any treatment at present.

The Organisation of the Programme

A number of questions about the organisation of the programme have to be asked before it can begin. Will the patient be treated individually or in a group? Will the programme run at home, in a side-room, or as part of the ward routine? Will any special equipment be required? Who will run the programme and who will supervise it? Emphasis has been given so far to the systematic assessment of the patient's problems. In the next two chapters various behaviour-change techniques will be discussed. However, although reliable assessment and appropriate behaviour-change techniques are essential for a successful programme, the treatment may fail if it is not organised well.

Repucci and Saunders[2] have emphasised the role of organisational support in the success of behavioural programmes. Programmes in institutions often fail, not because of faulty programming, but because insufficient attention is paid to the practical problems which can occur when a new model of care or treatment is introduced. These problems are listed in Table 6.1.

Many nurses see *bureaucracy* as mere 'red tape' or petty rules and regulations. However, red tape can stifle any new concept of care and is certainly not a problem peculiar to behaviour therapy. Care should always be taken to avoid breaking established rules without first getting some clearance to do so. Mealtimes which have to be altered, staff rotas adapted, or even patients allowed a long lie in bed on Sunday, may antagonise some 'bureaucrat' and may cause more than mere bad feeling. *Politics*, or political interference, may be a natural consequence of bureaucracy. If people believe, rightly or wrongly, that they have the

Table 6.1: Organisational Problems in the Clinical Setting

Buraucracy: rules, regulations and 'red tape' hinder the development of the programme.

Politics: approval or support for aspects of the programme are withheld or withdrawn, directly or indirectly.

Language: the aims or methods of the programme may be misinterpreted or mismanaged by staff who do not understand the technical language.

Staff: nurses, and other support staff, can sabotage the programme — intentionally or by accident — and must be managed carefully.

Resources: inadequate supplies of personnel, materials or appropriate treatment settings can handicap the programme.

Ideology: staff with competing philosophies about care and treatment may feel threatened by the behavioural model.

Personality: the nurse must be able to sell the approach to her colleagues and perhaps the patient.

Compromise: the practical restrictions of the treatment setting will demand that the final programme is a slimline version of the original plan.

sole right to give permission for changes, or to approve programmes, grave difficulties may arise if they are ignored. The peculiar *language* of behaviourism can become a handicap if all staff do not share the meaning intended. This is particularly so where common words or phrases assume a technical meaning. *Staff* are an obvious area of concern, since they can expedite or sabotage any programme, either wittingly or accidentally. The model of care and treatment presented by the *ideology* of behaviourism is not shared by everyone, especially in the larger teaching hospitals where it may compete with many other 'schools of thought'. The nurse should be aware that others may hold quite different views about how the mentally ill or handicapped should be nursed and that the behavioural approach may be seen as a threat to their independence. *Resources* are another crucial issue. If the programme depends heavily on money, staff or facilities, then it will be disrupted if these are withdrawn or not supplied. The *personality* of the nurse is important since she may be required to 'sell' the behavioural model, either to the patient or to her colleagues. If she is not a good salesperson then a good scheme may be devalued. Finally it is evident that changes in care or treatment policies occur gradually, if not at snail's pace. Most treatment proposals begin as an ideal and are whittled down by the considerations illustrated above, often to a mere shadow of their former selves. Although *compromise* is part of the reality of care-planning, the nurse should guard against ending up with a programme which may be the opposite of what she first intended.

The Planner and Presenter. This book is aimed at the nurse who will plan and conduct behavioural programmes. She may be an enrolled nurse on a hospital ward or a clinical specialist with a roving commission over several hospitals and community clinics. Where a nurse is planning programmes to be carried out by nurses under her supervision, she will assume the role of *planner*, the person with the knowledge.[3] The nurses running the programme, the therapeutic team, are the programme *presenters* and are those with the best opportunity to help the patient change his behaviour. In Brian's case his mother might present all, or part, of the programme when he is at home. Mrs Smith's mother might also carry out some aspect of her daughter's treatment under the guidance of, for example, the community nurse. The following guidelines aim to ensure that the planner meets the needs of the presenters as well as those of the patient.[4]

Making a Start. Where the nurse is planning a behavioural programme in a new situation she should select nurses who will be supportive and should avoid those who are resistant to new ideas. To enlist and maintain such support it is advisable to:

(1) Begin with a simple *demonstration* of the value of behaviour therapy.
(2) Work only with the resources available, leaving requests for more money, staff, equipment, etc., until the approach has proven itself.
(3) Work only with small groups of patients or individuals. The larger the group, the greater the strain on the nursing team.
(4) Train only those nurses who will be key staff in the programme.

Managing the Team. The ideal goal is to cultivate a small team which will be motivated to plan and develop their own programmes. A team which is encouraged by their own results will find added enthusiasm for their work and will require less supervision. This goal can be achieved by:

(1) Ensuring that each nurse knows *what* she is meant to do, *how* she is meant to do it and *what to do* if complications occur.
(2) Arranging brief but regular meetings to discuss achievements as well as problems.
(3) Avoiding situations where the team will be criticised harshly or unfairly. The planner should act as a 'troubleshooter' dealing with any complaints and preventing loss of morale.
(4) Asking significant people, e.g. senior nursing staff, tutors etc., to give encouragement to the team.

Siting the Programme.   When behaviour therapy is established as part of an overall policy, programmes should be set up where the patient's need is greatest, not simply to make life easier for staff or management. To ensure this the planner should:

(1) Avoid working with staff who have failed to respond to change in the past.
(2) Avoid working in facilities which are inadequate or which have obstructed developments in the past.
(3) Encourage staff to see the programme as a way of extending their present expertise and effectiveness, not as a criticism or demonstration of their inadequacy.

Liaison.   No nurse is an island. The planner, in particular, relies upon the support of a range of people: administrators, clinicians and educationalists. She should ensure that good communications are maintained at all times. This can be achieved by:

(1) Asking for *advice* about resources, trends or policies.
(2) Asking for *help* when problems are met, e.g. staffing, finances.
(3) Inviting senior staff, from all professions, to discuss the development of behavioural programmes, on a regular basis.

Stress Management.   Behavioural programmes can be source of stress for all staff involved. To reduce this the planner should:

(1) Make the role of each nurse specific and unambiguous.
(2) Communicate directly, and *informally*, with the team on all matters concerning their role and responsibilities. Formality encourages stress and may cause staff to hide fears or anxieties.
(3) Discuss all doubts or problems as soon as they occur.

Table 6.2: Key Factors in the Organisation of a Therapeutic Unit

Regular staff meetings	— mutual support within team; opportunity for problem-solving.
Simple record format	— details of patient's problems, assets and aims of treatment readily available to all staff.
Patient allocation	— consistent support for each patient: increases focus on the individual.
In-service training	— basic clinical skills necessary to operate programme; regular up-dating of skills and knowledge.
Operational policy	— clear perspective of role for individual nurse; overall appreciation of function of unit.

(4) Encourage the team to work together. This cohesion will offset the danger of isolation of individual members.

Durham[5] has suggested that these insurance policies can be built around a simple organisational skeleton (see Table 6.2). Regular meetings can be used to preview plans and review progress. Staff also have the opportunity to acknowledge difficulties and gain the support of colleagues in solving problems. Such meetings should be open to the whole team and all decisions recorded.

All staff need a simple record-keeping format, one which describes the patient's problems, assets, aims of treatment and how they are to be achieved. This should also include a *problem list*, details of treatment *plans* and a record of decisions made at meetings. This will enable new or temporary staff to become acquainted with the patient's care and management.

Patient allocation ensures that every patient receives regular support and attention. This will promote accountability for implementing individual programmes, encouraging a sense of achievement, responsibility and purpose. This also allows each patient one nurse to act as his 'advocate' when such help is needed.

Training, as noted earlier, should be geared to staff in key roles. Where possible staff should be kept abreast of new techniques, although all training should be aimed at establishing clinical skills.

Durham also emphasises the value of an operational policy. This provides staff with a clear expectation of *their* role, whilst giving them an understanding of the overall functioning of the ward, unit or team. This document should describe the function of a ward, admission policy, routines, organisation and therapeutic approach and makes the entry of new staff much easier. Durham suggests that this should be written by the team, rather than imposed upon them.

Selection of Appropriate Techniques

In many medical settings the *prescription* of treatment is a straight-forward affair. Although specific behavioural techniques can be recommended for certain problems, a wide range of interventions are often possible. In many cases a number of techniques will be amalgamated into a treatment package. In Chapters 7 and 8 'overt' and 'covert' change techniques are described. When selecting an appropriate technique the nurse must take account of the nature of the problem, where treatment will take place and the likelihood that the patient will respond to this method. She must ensure not only that the technique has a good 'track record', but that it will be suitable for this patient in this situation.

Many studies are published every year comparing and contrasting the effectiveness of different methods in treating specific problems. The nurse should try to select a technique which is supported by some recent research. Although it is impossible to read every report in every journal, the nurse should guard against assuming that, because techniques were once popular and highly recommended, their value is beyond question.[6,7]

The treatment situation is also important. Where programmes have to be run in situations which are far from ideal, treatment techniques must be selected carefully. For instance, incontinence might be treated best by the 'rapid toiletting' method.[8] However, the demands on the nurse's time and energy are severe under this system, even if only for a short time. If staff are unfamiliar with the system, or if adequate numbers of nurses to carry out programme cannot be guaranteed, then this approach may be 'inappropriate'. Similarly, some techniques, aimed at reducing behaviour, can be successful in controlled studies, but may be inappropriate in some clinical situations. Where reinforcement is 'withdrawn' or 'withheld' the nurse may spend most of her time waiting to implement the treatment. Some treatment methods emphasise treating the patient in his natural situation. This may be impossible if the nurse cannot go to the patient, or if he has been admitted to hospital. As in the examples above, a treatment technique must be found to suit the patient *and* his new situation.

A third consideration is the patient himself and his view of the treatment. Even highly successful techniques are suitable only for certain patients. In Chapter 8, covert methods are described; these depend upon the patient's ability to communicate and to use his powers of memory, fantasy and thought, etc. In general these methods are inappropriate for patients like Sally and Brian. However, these methods can be adapted to suit mentally handicapped people and some psychiatric patients with more severe problems of living,[9] providing that the technique is adapted to suit the individual patient.

In the same vein it is often assumed that all people with the same problem will respond to the same techniques. Desensitisation is a commonly used technique for phobias. However where this technique is used in imagination, only those patients who are able to imagine the scenes described will have a chance of responding successfully. Other techniques, which involve the patient in studying his own behaviour, anticipating certain events and adopting certain thinking strategies, all hinge upon the patient's ability to use certain mental processes. It is clear that many patients do not have sufficient control over these processes to benefit from such techniques, even patients with normal intelligence and no serious mental disorder. In every case the initial assessment should indicate whether or not the patient will benefit from such techniques. If not, then some alternative must be found.

Patients may also prove unresponsive to more overt behaviour-change methods. Many severaly handicapped children fail to respond to techniques based upon modelling or vicarious learning, through lack of attentional control or other 'mediational' processes. Punishment-based techniques may stimulate violent reactions which may be worse than the problem the nurse is trying to solve. Where patients are unresponsive or 'sensitive' to certain techniques, some alternative must be sought.

Finally, the technique which appears to offer the best solution may be unacceptable to the patient. For instance, reports show that *flooding* can be a quick and lasting solution to certain anxiety/avoidance problems. However, the patient may refuse to spend long periods in a situation which he fears greatly, in spite of the benefits promised to him. Similarly, many patients drop out of treatment because they do not like their 'role' in the therapy programme. For example, patients may feel embarrassed when asked to role-play situations in an assertion training group. Some patients may find this worse than their presenting problem and may discontinue treatment. In both examples, the nurse should be sensitive to the patient's views. After all he is the consumer.

In a similar vein, staff may find certain techniques unpalatable and may be unwilling to carry them out. This is well-documented in situations where aversive methods are used.[10] In such cases the nurse must decide whether to change the technique or to change the staff – or their views – in order that the original plan may proceed.

The Evaluation

Evaluation is part of the treatment programme rather than a stage in itself. Three kinds of evaluation, or judgement, are made in the course of therapy. The nurse judges:

(1) The value of the baseline information. What is the effect of different observers? How reliable are they and how valid are the observational methods used?
(2) Whether or not the behaviour has changed in the direction intended during intervention.
(3) Whether these improvements last, when treatment is discontinued. In this case a follow-up measure would be taken perhaps some months after the first intervention.

These evaluations involve repetition of the same measures across baseline, intervention and follow-up stages. A fourth kind of evaluation is possible. This involves judging whether or not the techniques used were responsible for the changes which have occurred. Evaluation of the fourth kind is important since it adds to our knowledge about the patient and may prove useful in helping patients with similar problems.

Research Designs.   Evaluation of this fourth kind is achieved by use of research designs. The simplest of these is the A-B design, where A represents the baseline and B the intervention phase. Measures taken during each phase are compared and if an appropriate change in frequency, or duration, etc., occurs, the programme is judged a success and the techniques used given a major share of the credit. This design is weak since many other factors could have helped effect the change.[11]

The A-B-A-B design, often called the reversal, tries to answer the questions prompted by the A-B design. Once again A represents baseline and B the intervention. After a period of intervention the treatment is stopped and the baseline conditions reinstituted. After a period of 'reversal' the treatment is reapplied. If the behaviour does not change in accordance with the introduction and removal of the treatment conditions, then some other factor must be influencing the behaviour.

Figure 6.8: Reversal Design

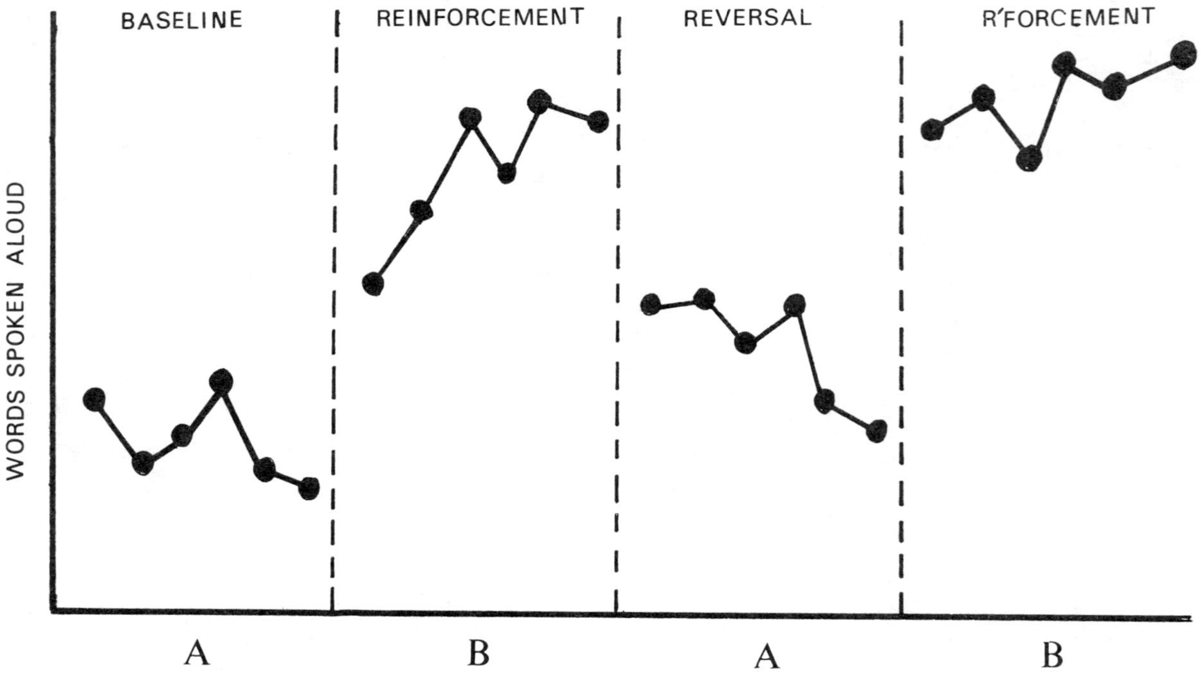

Figure 6.8 shows a reversal design. When the intervention stops, the behaviour returns to near the original baseline level. When the treatment is reapplied the the behaviour increases in frequency, suggesting that the technique used is responsible for the change taking place.

Problems in Using Reversal Designs.   There are three main problems associated with the use of reversal designs. First, it may be argued that it is undesirable to restore a patient's behaviour to the baseline, even for a short period. This would be the case for any self-injurious or aggressive behaviour, where most people would be satisfied to see a change in behaviour which *appeared* to be the result of the intervention employed. Secondly, changes in behaviour may be effected initially by the treatment programme, but may soon come under the control of some other factor. For instance, a child may be punished each time he is aggressive towards his peer group. As his aggressive behaviour decreases he has the opportunity to engage in more positive interactions with other children. If a reversal were introduced now, the behaviour would be unlikely to return to the baseline level, since more appropriate behaviour, maintained by peer-group reinforcement, has taken its place. Where skills training is the focus of the programme, reversals are also inappropriate. Even when the training programme is withdrawn, it is unlikely that the person will 'unlearn' the newly acquired skill.

Multiple Baseline Design.   The multiple baseline offers an alternative to the reversal. Here a number of behaviours are measured under baseline conditions. One of these is selected for intervention, the rest remaining under the original baseline conditions (see Figure 6.9). If the treatment condition is controlling the behaviour it will change only the behaviour selected for intervention, the rest remaining at their baseline level. The effectiveness of any treatment technique can be evaluated by observing its effect upon a range of behaviours, treated in strict sequence. This sequence may parallel the list of targets drawn up for the treatment programme.

Ethical Considerations

Throughout this chapter the terms *change* and *change techniques* have been used regularly. However the concept of change, especially where it is *engineered* systematically by nurses or other therapists, invokes a number of moral considerations. It can be argued that behaviour therapy may give the patient a degree of mastery over his personal problems which would not be possible by other approaches. Where the

Figure 6.9: Multiple Baseline Design — Percentage of 'Successes'

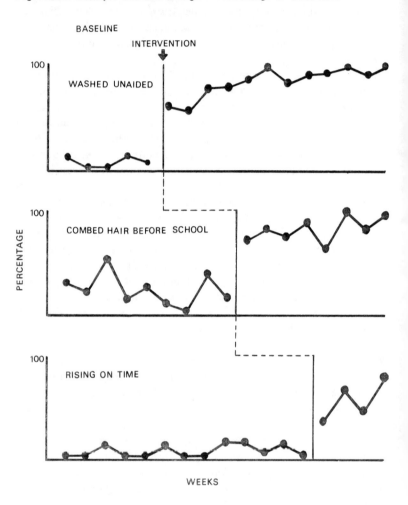

patient learns to control excesses, or acquires new skills, restrictions previously imposed upon him may be lifted. Whether this involves regained continence or increased assertiveness, the change may extend the patient's personal freedom. Behaviour therapy also offers some patients the chance to participate in their treatment or even to treat themselves. Efforts are also made to reduce the patient's dependence upon his 'therapist'; this may help restore the dignity of a person who has been demoralised by his problems of living.

In spite of these arguments in favour of behaviour therapy, many critics would suggest that the behavioural approach restricts the patient's freedom and may remove his dignity altogether.[12] Ethical arguments, for and against behaviourism, are too diverse for summary here. In Appendix 3 some practical advice, regarding the planning of behavioural programmes, is provided. These guidelines do not argue any philosophical case. Instead they suggest ways of ensuring that the patient is protected from treatment systems which are ill-conceived or contrary to the wishes of the patient or his advocate.

The major ethical questions raised by *any* behaviour-change programme, whether behavioural or not, are as follows:

(1) Who decides what is normal?
(2) How can we ensure that treatment is based upon a realistic assessment of the patient's problems?
(3) Should we change the patient's situation, rather than his behaviour?
(4) How can we ensure that we are using the best therapeutic techniques and are evaluating treatment reliably and objectively?

Does the Patient Need Treatment? The nurse must question whether treatment is in the patient's best interests or if someone else will benefit from the change in his behaviour. Even where a patient volunteers for treatment, he may be influenced heavily by family, care staff or the subtler forces of public opinion. We must consider the extent to which the patient's agreement to accept treatment is a 'free choice'.

Patients may also ask for treatment which will infringe the rights of others. In helping Mrs Smith cope better with her mother, should we take the mother's feelings into account? Should we help an alcoholic reduce his anxiety and depression which he suffers each time he assaults his wife and children or should we help him to stop beating up his family? It is often suggested that, where informed consent is given, no ethical problems are involved. However, even if the patient feels that a certain kind of treatment is right for him, the nurse must decide if she should help him. Where informed consent cannot be given, as in Brian's and Sally's cases, someone should attempt to speak for the patient and to serve his best interests.

The Goals of Therapy. Any treatment programme should set realistic goals, acknowledging the patient's current level of functioning and ability to change. Progress through the stages of therapy should be paced, to minimise failure and stress. The patient should be retained at any one stage of the programme only for as long as is necessary. Programmes can fossilise all too easily into routines which become an end in themselves.

The programme should also offer therapeutic benefits which outweigh any emotional costs involved. Where feared situations are presented to phobic patients, desired objects withdrawn from children, or painful stimuli — such as shocks, noise or reprimands — used, the nurse should be confident that the benefits which the patient will gain will cancel out most of the unpleasantness involved. It has been suggested that the ethical justification for any technique lies in the value of the outcome *relative* to the severity or undesirability of the procedure itself.[13] Amputation to cure a hangnail would be unethical, but might be essential to solve the problem of gangrene.

Programmes which use positive reinforcement do not escape these ethical dilemmas. This is especially the case where the patient is deprived, even temporarily, of positive reinforcement which was once freely available. It is often argued that any reinforcement used in such situations should be over and above that which is the patient's *by right*. Often, the problem is to establish what are the patient's rights.

In some cases parents, relatives and care staff may be part of the patient's problem. It may be necessary to encourage them to change their behaviour towards the patient, either to resolve the problem directly or to maintain some change which has taken place. Patients are often treated successfully in hospital, only to have the problem 're-instituted' when they return to their original environment. One of the goals of treatment must be to try to change the patient's *relationships* with such 'significant others'.

Determinism and Choice.   It is often argued that no ethical dilemma will arise providing that the patient, or someone who speaks for him, makes the major decisions about treatment goals and the methods to be used. This viewpoint reduces the person directing the treatment to that of a mere technician, someone who merely *enables* the patient to reach his desired objective. Mahoney suggests that since behaviourism argues that the patient's values and beliefs stem from previous learning *and* current influences, this is an ironic viewpoint.[14] The patient's views about treatment, etc., cannot be 'determined' *and* 'free' at the same time. Indeed it is naive to suggest that nurses, and other health care staff, can leave their values and prejudices behind, when they enter into a 'therapy contract' with a patient. Mahoney suggests that the only realistic course of action is for all of us to make our value biases known to the patient or his advocate, wherever appropriate. Once the patient or his advocate is aware of out view of the problem, he should be helped to make his own evaluation of the problem and any possible solution. Although we have 'come clean' in terms of how we see the situation, we may still be steering the patient or his advocate in the direction we think he ought to go. In many cases we may *engineer* the patient without being aware that we are doing so. If the values of the patient and the nurse are extremely polarised and might make the establishment of a therapeutic relationship difficult, someone with less radically different views should be nominated to work with the patient.

Summary

Any treatment programme begins with the baseline. From this a picture of the patient and his problems emerges, which provides the basis for planning the treatment strategy. The final stage of the assessment involves translating the assessment information into a more 'readable' format, often a graph or chart which nurse and patient can study together and use to monitor progress. This translation heralds the first stage of the programme design. Using the baseline data the nurse can ask the important questions concerning treatment goals, the commencement date, the organisation and evaluation of the programme, the treatment methods and any ethical implications which might be raised by the whole exercise.

Where the treatment programme involves only patient and therapist, the design issues are largely technical ones; the nurse must find a treatment format which suits her and the patient. Where other staff, or the patient's relatives, are involved, the programme design stage may become more complex. The treatment programme in the hospital setting often needs to be a more open-ended affair, allowing for inputs from other professionals and from other treatment models. Although the programme may be straightforward, its organisation and presentation may be complex.

In some situations the nurse may be able to use a standardised treatment programme, which requires only minor adaptations to suit the patient concerned. In other situations she may need to devise a treatment format which is unique and may suit no other patient. If the nurse is fortunate, she may find a ready-made solution to her patient's problem or someone willing to construct one for her. In many situations she will find that no such instant answer is available and will need to prepare and test several possible answers herself. (Appendix 4 shows a checklist used to monitor the treatment programme, in a hospital setting, from the receipt of the referral to follow-up.)

Notes

1. A film by Ivor Lovaas is a particularly dramatic illustration of the success of highly intensive therapy. See: Lovaas, O.I. *Reinforcement Therapy*, 16 mm sound film (Philadelphia, Smith Kline & French Laboratories, 1966).

2. Repucci, N.D. and Saunders, J.T. 'Social psychology of behaviour modification: problems of implementation in natural settings', *American Psychologist* (September 1976), pp. 649–60.

3. This concept was originally proposed by Tharp, R.G. and Wetzel, R.J. *Behaviour Modification in the Natural Environment* (New York, Academic Press, 1969).

4. These guidelines are influenced by the work of Georgiades, N.J. and Phillimore, L. 'The myth of the hero-innovator and alternative strategies for organizational change'. In: C.C. Kiernan and F.P. Woodward (eds), *Behaviour Modification with the Severely Retarded* (New York, Association of Scientific Publishers, 1975).

5. Durham, R. Personal communication.

6. Barker, P., Docherty, P. and Hird, J. ' "Showing an improvement": an examination of variables central to the token economy system', *International Journal of Nursing Studies*, vol. 17 (1980), pp. 25–37.

7. Fraser, D. 'Critical variables in the token economy system', *Behavioural Psychotherapy*, vol. 6 (1978), pp. 46–55.

8. Azrin, N.H. and Foxx, R.M. 'A rapid method of toilet training the institutionally retarded', *Journal of Applied Behaviour Analysis*, vol. 4 (1971), pp. 89–99.

9. See: Meichenbaum, D.H. and Cameron, R. 'Training schizophrenics to talk to themselves: a means of developing attentional controls', *Behaviour Therapy*, vol. 4 (1973), pp. 515–34.

10. Problems associated with the use of aversive procedures are described in Chapter 8 of Rimm, D.C. and Masters, J.C. *Behaviour Therapy: Techniques and Empirical Findings* (New York, Academic Press, 1979).

11. See: Hersen, M. and Barlow, D.H. *Single Case Experimental Designs: Strategies for Studying Behaviour Change* (New York, Pergamon, 1976).

12. For a general discussion, see: Barker, P. 'Ethics, nursing and behaviour modification', *Nursing Times* (29 May 1980).

13. This view is taken from a short article by Cahoon, D.D. 'Balancing procedures against outcomes', *Hospital and Community Psychiatry* (July 1968), pp. 228–9.

14. Mahoney, M.J. *Cognition and Behaviour Modification* (Cambridge, Mass., Ballinger, 1974), p. 284.

CHANGING BEHAVIOUR FROM THE OUTSIDE

A poem is what happens when an anxiety meets a technique.
— Laurence Durrell

Behaviour Control and Behaviour Change

Behaviour does not occur in a vacuum. All behaviour is under the 'control' of the events which surround us, whether subtle or more obvious. However, although this assertion is typically 'behaviourist', there is still some disagreement, within behaviourism, as to the meaning of the term 'control'. As far as nurses are concerned it is important only to appreciate that our behaviour is inextricably linked to the events which go on around us. The extent to which our behaviour is 'self-willed' or 'automatic' is unclear and appears to depend greatly upon the situation and the behaviour concerned. However, before we consider the idea of attempting to change a patient's behaviour, we should attempt to understand 'why' he is showing particular patterns of behaviour at present.

What is the nature of his problem? Would it be solved by increasing or decreasing existing behaviour or does he need to learn some new skill? What conditions appear to control the problem behaviour? Does the problem behaviour have any effect upon the patient's environment? What effect does it have upon the patient?

Answers to these questions will help us decide upon an appropriate change technique: one which will bring the behaviour under a new form of 'control'. This may be a form of patient-directed 'self-control' or another kind of environmental control. If all behaviour is under some kind of control already, then the aim of behaviour therapy is to bring it under a more adaptive form of control. As Skinner has argued:

> Dependence on things is not independence. The child who does not need to be told that it is time to go to school has come under the control of more subtle and more useful stimuli. The child who has learned what to say and how to behave in getting along with other people is under the control of social contingencies. People who get along well under the mild contingencies of approval and disapproval are controlled as effectively (and in many ways more effectively than) the citizens of a police state. Orthodoxy controls through the

establishment of rules, but the mystic is no freer because the contingencies which have shaped his behaviour are more personal or
idiosyncratic. Those who work productively because of the reinforcing value of what they produce are under the sensitive and
powerful control of the products. Those who learn in the natural
environment are under a form of control as powerful as any control
exerted by a teacher.[1]

In this chapter we shall discuss some ways in which we can increase
or decrease more overt patterns of behaviour, in an attempt to teach
the patient new ways of living. By using these techniques the nurse is
acting as a kind of teacher, helping the patient establish a new, more
adaptive, form of control over his behaviour. As Skinner has argued, the
role of the teacher is akin to that of nature. Although the techniques
which we shall now discuss are technical and artificial, they are based
upon our assumptions about the 'natural laws' which govern behaviour.

Techniques which change behaviour 'from the outside' depend
heavily upon the manipulation of events in the patient's environment.
These may occur in one of three ways:

(1) Changes can be arranged by the nurse. In this situation the nurse
    applies the change-techniques *to* the patient.
(2) Changes can be arranged by nurse and patient together, both
    collaborating in the delivery of the technique.
(3) Changes can be arranged by the patient. The nurse's role here is
    to teach the patient how to apply these techniques to himself.

Therapist-controlled Techniques

Positive Reinforcement

A number of techniques which increase behaviour are built around the
concept of positive reinforcement. This is usually defined as any event
which, when it follows a behaviour, increases the likelihood of that
behaviour being repeated in the future. Although it is often confused
with 'reward', positive reinforcement does not always subscribe to the
common view that rewards are pleasant or aesthetic events. Some
people like to be complimented on their looks, whereas others find
such comments embarrassing. Some people love chocolate, others
loathe it. Some children shun the cuddles and caresses which other
children enjoy, while masochists (or sportsmen) seem to enjoy what

most of us would call self-inflicted pain. Positive reinforcement is highly individual: one man's meat may be another man's poison. Any behaviour which is positively reinforced will be strengthened. If a withdrawn patient is reinforced each time he speaks, this will increase the likelihood that he will speak in the furure. The patient's speech will be strengthened in much the same way that a concrete pillar is reinforced by the steel bars within it.

The Reinforcement Survey.   Our assessment of the patient should include a detailed list of his reinforcers. Some of these will be highly prized or greatly detested, whereas others will be less potent. Our reinforcement survey involves giving the patient a free choice and discovering which things or situations he selects, avoids or rejects. A number of questionnaires have been developed to identify positive and negative reinforcers.[2,3] Where he cannot complete these himself, the nurse would discuss the questions with the patient or complete the survey from her own knowledge of the patient. Where the patient is unable to speak, simple reinforcement tests may be set up, so that he can show which things attract or repel him. Our functional analysis should give us some idea of what factors reinforce specific patterns of behaviour. By showing particular patterns of behaviour the patient may gain something he likes, or avoid or postpone something which he finds unpleasant or aversive.

Conditioned Reinforcement.   Reinforcers can be *primary* (e.g. food, drink, warmth) or *secondary* (e.g. money, possessions, compliments). Secondary reinforcers are learned, whereas primary reinforcers are natural. Although secondary reinforcers could be called the luxuries of life, they are often what makes life worth living for most of us. The token economy system uses a special kind of conditioned reinforcer. Here the patient learns to associate tokens, either plastic discs, paper notes, or punchmarks on a card, with a 'back-up reinforcer'. Although at first worthless, the token acquires reinforcing properties through association with the back-up reinforcer. The patient may prize the tokens in the same way as we value the coins and notes of our currency.

The token economy is based upon the Premack Principle. This states that any high-probability behaviour (HPB) which is contingent upon a low-probability behaviour (LPB) will reinforce the low-rate behaviour. Sally spends much of her day sitting in the dayroom smoking (HPBs). She is loathe to wash herself or tidy her bedroom (LPBs). If arrangements were made that she could only smoke or use the dayroom armchairs *after* she has groomed herself and tidied her room, the HPBs would increase and strengthen her grooming and domestic behaviour.

In many cases it is impractical to try to reinforce one behaviour with another in this fashion. A patient may fail to associate 'attending therapy on Monday morning' and 'going into town' on a Saturday afternoon. Tokens are often used to bridge the gap between the target and the reinforcing behaviour. When the token is given it acts as a signal that the patient will be able to engage in some choice behaviour later in the day or next week, etc.[4]

Building New Patterns of Behaviour.   Positive reinforcement is used to increase the frequency or duration of behaviours which are already an established part of the patient's repertoire, no matter how small. However, where the target behaviour is not already part of the patient's repertoire, it will be necessary to help the patient show the desired behaviour, so that it can be reinforced. A variety of *prompts*[5] are used to ensure that the target behaviour occurs in the appropriate situation. Once the behaviour is established the prompts can be *faded*, or phased out systematically, leaving the person to show the behaviour as a response to the natural cues of the situation. These may be gross or minimal, depending upon the amount of help required to ensure that the behaviour is shown. Prompting and reinforcement could be combined in Brian's case, to help teach him to sit on a chair. If telling him what to do (verbal prompt) was unsuccessful, then the nurse could signal the request – waving and pointing towards the seat (gestural prompt). If this failed she would guide him towards the seat (physical prompt), gesturing and instructing him at the same time. Once Brian is able to sit down with maximum prompting, the nurse will give less and less physical assistance until he performs the behaviour with only gestural and verbal prompting. These prompts will be faded gradually until he sits under instruction and finally in response to the natural stimulus of the seat and the situation (e.g. dining room or classroom).

Prompting and reinforcement can be used to establish a response to a specific stimulus. In the example above all the cues, or prompts, are related to 'seat' and 'sitting'. The child is reinforced as soon as he sits on the seat, thereby strengthening 'sitting on a seat', as opposed to sitting on a table or the floor, etc. Many behaviour patterns must be shown in response to only one kind of stimulus. Although any toilet could be used to teach Brian the basics of toilet use, the skill is not complete until he can tell a 'male' toilet from a 'female' one. Teaching people to sit, stand, walk into, sleep on, or talk to one thing or person *and not another*, is called *discrimination training*. Although this is practised most often with children or mentally handicapped people, socially inexperienced or naive people – like Mrs Smith – may also have difficulty in making much finer discriminations, e.g. 'sizing up' social situations, 'knowing what is appropriate behaviour' in different situations. Alternatively, some people need *generalisation training*: they need to learn how to show the same behaviour in response to different situational cues. A patient may follow one nurse's instructions, but ignore all the other nurses. A child may speak freely at home, but may be 'shy' in other people's homes. Generalisation training involves a gradual introduction of 'new' stimuli, to which the patient does not respond at present, and reinforcement for responding, even minimally, to each new situation.

Many behaviour problems involve inappropriate stimulus control. People who urinate or undress in the street, kiss total strangers or tell blue jokes at a cocktail party, may be over-generalising their behaviour and may need to discriminate more carefully. Patients who speak in a social-skills group but withdraw on return to the ward, or who work diligently at school but 'forget' to do their homework, need to generalise their behaviour to a wider range of situations.

Much of our everyday behaviour involves complex chains or sequences of behaviour, rather than single actions. Speaking, dressing, using the toilet, boarding a bus, etc., are made up of a number of different behaviours closely linked to form a pattern of behaviour. Where the patient cannot perform the whole chain of behaviour this will need to be built up gradually, reinforcing successive approximations of the final target behaviour. This *shaping* technique resembles a moulding action. The behaviour is 'shaped' in the way that a sculptor moulds his final image from a lump of clay. Although the original behaviour bears little resemblance to the final target, as it is 'shaped' through the successive stages it becomes more and more like the final target response. In an early experiment, Isaacs[6] shaped speech in a 'mute' patient by reinforcing at first any eye movements towards the therapist, then any small movements of the lips, and then any spontaneous sounds, no matter how small, such as coughing or clearing his throat. Finally these sounds were shaped gradually into actual vocalisation, in the form of parts of words and then full words and sentences,

Behaviours such as dressing or making a bed involve selecting, holding, moving around and finally putting down or letting go, in a carefully controlled sequence. *Backward chaining* is a technique which can be used to ensure that these complex chains are learned quickly.

Instead of teaching the patient to perform the behaviour 'from the beginning', the process is reversed. The nurse prompts the patient through each step in the chain, leaving him to complete the very last part, e.g. smoothing out the wrinkles in a bedcover, or pulling his jumper over the top of his trousers. Although the patient is only a passive participant throughout the steps in the chain, he completes the final movement and is reinforced for 'completing the behaviour'. At the next stage he is asked to complete the last two stages in the chain before being reinforced and so on *backwards* through the chain until he can begin and proceed to the completion of the behaviour unaided.[7]

Considerations in the Use of Reinforcement

Contingency.   Reinforcement should always be delivered *contingent* upon the target behaviour; a clear relationship should exist between the patient's behaviour and the events which follow. Where non-communicative patients are concerned it may be advisable to make this contingent relationship clear by giving the reinforcement *as soon as* the behaviour occurs. Where the patient can discuss his programme, reinforcement may be delayed if this is an advantage. If a patient can associate a compliment with his grooming earlier in the day, then the compliment will reinforce the grooming, no matter how far apart the two events are. If he cannot make such a connection, then each act of washing, combing hair, etc., may need to be reinforced as it occurs.

Satiation Effects.   When we are hungry, food is a very potent reinforcer. After we have eaten, food loses its appeal and may become aversive if forced upon us. Now we would prefer other reinforcers, such as a cigarette or a drink. *Satiation* occurs when the patient has 'had enough' of the reinforcer, whether it is food, drink or a television programme. In order to overcome this problem the programme should accommodate a range of reinforcers, so that a 'new' reinforcer can be substituted when satiation is reached. Some conditioned reinforcers, like money, tokens and social approval, may be highly resistant to satiation. Since money and tokens can be 'stored' for future use and social reinforcement 'evaporates' as soon as it is given, these should be given a central role in the programme, if appropriate.

Food and Drink Reinforcers.   Sweets, snacks, drinks and parts of complete meals have been used widely to build up behaviour in mentally handicapped[8,9] and psychotic patients[10]. These primary reinforcers should be used only with patients who are not amenable to other forms of reinforcement. Apart from the ethical objections to the use of such a basic right as food, other problems may develop.

(1) Food and drink are only effective if the patient is hungry or thirsty to some extent. This means that restrictions must be imposed upon the availability of food and drink, outwith the programme.
(2) The use of food and drink may cause or exacerbate problems of obesity or dental caries or may interfere with normal appetite.
(3) Unless the reinforcer is 'rationed' very carefully, satiation may build up very quickly, even within one sesssion.
(4) Eating or drinking may interfere with some behaviours, such as speech training programmes or where the hands must be used.
(5) Where the nurse is working with two or three patients, with different reinforcement preferences, she may have great difficulty handling and carrying the reinforcers. This problem is heightened where prompts have to be given, equipment operated and observations made and recorded.

Social Reinforcement.   Praise, attention, kissing, cuddling, nodding, winking, smiling, etc., can all be social reinforcers. They can be delivered quickly and easily, to a group as easily as one person. Although social reinforcement is not subject to the same satiation effects as primary reinforcers, the patient may tire of repeated compliments, nodding or other signs of 'approval'. Social reinforcement is more appropriate and dignified, than the manipulation of basic reinforcers. However, if social reinforcement is not given with enthusiasm, conviction or sincerity, the patient may find it aversive. Primary reinforcers may be given successfully by a machine or a robot. Social reinforcement is dependent upon the medium of a warm, friendly and genuine human being.

Reinforcement Schedules.   If reinforcement is given continuously, each time the behaviour occurs, and then is withdrawn, the behaviour will stop. When we put money in a vending machine and nothing happens, we do not repeat the behaviour as the reinforcement expected was not forthcoming. To prevent this *extinction* occurring the reinforcement is 'thinned out' gradually, using reinforcement schedules.

In a *fixed ratio* schedule, reinforcement is given only after a certain number of behaviours have been performed. A child might be reinforced each time he puts one block on top of another (continuous reinforcement). Then he would be reinforced after building two, then three, then four blocks and so on. As the reinforcement is 'thinned out' the child performs more behaviour for the same amount of reinforcement.

In *variable ratio* schedules reinforcement is given at random: *on average* every two, three or ten times. The child might be given reinforcement after the eighth, sixteenth, thirtieth and fortieth 'block-building behaviours'. This would represent reinforcement on average every ten times, a variable ratio of ten. This schedule, which is used in gambling machines, makes behaviour very resistant to extinction. Since the patient is unaware of when the next unit of reinforcement will appear, he continues showing the behaviour in anticipation of reinforcement 'sooner or later'.

Reinforcement can also be thinned out across time, in the *fixed interval* and *variable interval* schedules. These are useful where the behaviour − such as speaking, or working − occurs across a wide time span. The first behaviour performed after the time interval is up, is reinforced. If a five-minute interval was selected the nurse would reinforce the first word spoken, step taken, or sentence written, after the five minutes is up. This schedule may be useful for nurses reinforcing patients playing games, working in occupational therapy or completing self-care routines. The weakness in the fixed interval is that the patient will be able to calculate when reinforcement is next due. He may well increase his behaviour in anticipation of its arrival. This can be overcome by adopting a variable schedule where the intervals are *on average* every five minutes etc.

Negative Reinforcement

Behaviour can also be strengthened by *negative* reinforcement. In this case the patient will perform some behaviour in order to escape from or avoid something unpleasant. Taking pain-killing drugs, switching off an alarm or hiding from an over-talkative neighbour, are all examples of negative reinforcement: we perform a specific behaviour to avoid or escape from something unpleasant.

Negative reinforcement has been used most widely with alcoholism, overeating and sexual deviance.[11] The patient is usually given electric shocks when viewing pictures of drinking, eating or sexually deviant situations. The shocks can be terminated by switching off the deviant image and replacing it with a more adaptive one, e.g. cup of tea, diet sheet, etc. However, any positive results gained under controlled treatment conditions often fail to generalise to the everyday situation. A similar approach has been used to 'shape up' appropriate play behaviour in severely self-destructive children.[12] Although negative reinforcement is not used widely in behavioural programmes, it is very common in everyday life. Much of our behaviour is the result of avoiding criticism, complaints or other forms of legal or social censure. Where escape and avoidance are included in behavioural programmes they should be used to show the patient how to cope with the circumstances of everyday life.

Decreasing Behaviour

Extinction. When reinforcement is withdrawn suddenly the behaviour will reduce in frequency and soon stop. This is akin to the extinction of a flame by removing the oxygen it needs to continue burning. If Sally is refused consistently, each time she asks for a cigarette, she will stop asking at some stage in the future. However, since her behaviour has been established for many years, it may be maintained on a variable schedule and will take a very long time to extinguish. Usually, the behaviour increases in frequency when the reinforcement is withdrawn. Providing that the reinforcement is not reintroduced, the behaviour will gradually decrease. This brief escalation of the problem can be disturbing and many people often conclude (prematurely) that 'it isn't working'.

Differential Reinforcement of Other Behaviour (DRO). In DRO reinforcement is withdrawn from one behaviour (extinction) and reallocated to any other behaviour (positive reinforcement). A crying child would be ignored and then picked up as soon as he stops crying and begins, for example, playing with his toys. In some cases an incompatible behaviour is selected, rather than any other behaviour. The child would be reinforced for smiling and ignored when crying; since smiling and crying are incompatible an increase in the former will produce a decrease in the latter.

Time out from Reinforcement. Behaviour can also be reduced by removing the patient from a reinforcing situation or taking reinforcement from him, for a period of time. A child's toy might be taken away for five minutes, a trip to town postponed for a week, or a nurse's attention withdrawn for a few seconds. After this period of time-out is over, reinforcement is returned. Short periods of time-out should be used at first. If this is unsuccessful, they can be increased gradually, until an effective level is reached.

Response Cost. Where reinforcement is withdrawn permanently the patient is 'fined' for showing certain behaviours. Toys, cigarettes, and tokens can all be forfeited. In response cost the patient can remain in the treatment situation and can choose to continue showing the offending behaviour — and suffer further response cost — or show more adaptive behaviour, which will bring positive reinforcement.

Punishment. In layman's terms, punishment usually means the application of something unpleasant or painful. In behaviour therapy any stimulus which, when it follows a behaviour, decreases the likelihood of it being repeated is, by definition, a punisher. Punishment is defined by its effect, rather than by its appearance. As we noted earlier, some people enjoy pain, whilst others find cuddles and caresses unpleasant. Punishment can be used in two ways: by applying positive reinforcement to excess, *satiation*; and by applying something which the patient finds unpleasant, *aversion*. In satiation, reinforcement is given until it is no longer enjoyable or until it becomes unpleasant. Ayllon[13] described a patient who hoarded towels in her room. The nurses increased the number of towels she was given each day, until she had over six hundred in her room. The patient then began bringing out the towels and stopped hoarding them altogether. In aversion an electric shock, loud noise or reprimand, etc., is delivered contingent upon the behaviour. In order for punishment to be effective there should be no opportunity for escape. The punishment should be introduced at a high intensity, otherwise the patient may get used to it, and it should be delivered for every occurrence of the problem behaviour.

Problems in the Use of Punishment. In this chapter we have paid only passing reference to punishment methods for two reasons. First, there appear to be more successful ways of reducing problem behaviour, than by simply 'knocking it out' and secondly a number of complications arise from the use of punishment methods.

(1) When the patient is punished, either by losing a favourite toy or receiving a reprimand, he may experience an emotional reaction which may weaken the effect of the punishment. He may be unresponsive until this emotional reaction disappears and will not benefit from any further learning opportunities given to him.

(2) Painful punishment is also likely to produce aggression. For people, as well as animals, aggression is an instinctive form of defence, which is often negatively reinforced by the removal of the aversive stimulus. Although most often seen in the use of electric shock, it is

not altogether unlikely that a patient might attack a nurse for removing his teddy bear or cigarettes.

(3) Punishment often leads to escape and avoidance. The patient may associate the punishment with the nurse who delivers it and may avoid her even in positive reinforcement situations.

(4) Punishment raises a number of ethical issues. These may be heightened for nurses who have always seen themselves as providers of tender loving care. Many nurses find the whole concept of punishment morally repugnant and may refuse to participate in its use.

Punishment is entirely about teaching the patient *what not to do*. It does not help him learn how to behave in a more appropriate or rewarding manner. For this, and for the reasons above, punishment should only be used in conjunction with some positive reinforcement system or as a last resort in truly intractable cases.

Collaborating with the Patient

Where the patient can discuss his problems with the nurse and suggest possible solutions, the treatment programme may become more of a joint effort. Although we often assume that mentally handicapped people or those with a severe psychiatric illness cannot help themselves to any great extent, often this is not the case. Each patient should be assessed to determine the extent to which he might participate in his own treatment.

Collaborative methods can be grouped under the following headings: *contingency contracting* techniques, those using *modelling* and those using *exposure.*

Contingency Contracting

The reinforcement and punishment techniques described earlier can be incorporated into a contract between the patient and his 'therapist' or between the patient and some 'significant others'. In contingency contracting a clear statement is given of 'what will happen' if the patient engages in, or fails to show, the target behaviour. The contract can be used to arrange positive reinforcement *or* punishment contingencies, depending upon whether behaviour is to be increased or decreased. The 'contract' is most useful where the patient may try to manipulate the nurse or significant other, in order to avoid the contingencies. This is often the case with children and their parents, or between husband and wife. The contract can also be useful with patients like Sally who are likely to forget a verbal agreement and who can be 'reminded' by the sight of the contract.

The Contract Ingredients. The contract usually contains the following elements:

(1) A clear definition of the target behaviour. This may be a target for reduction or increase, but should be observable so that each 'side' can see whether or not the aims of the contract have been met.

(2) Clear details of the positive reinforcement each side expects to get from the contractual arrangement. The patient may expect to have a choice of television programmes, or the use of a favourite armchair. Nursing staff may expect him to do 'household chores' or attend the occupational therapy.

(3) Clear details of 'punishment' contingencies for failure to comply with the contract. In addition to the forfeiture of the positive reinforcers (2, above) existing reinforcers may be withdrawn or additional work given.

(4) Special bonuses may be arranged to provide incentives to maintain the targets over a long period of time. These bonuses may be 'scheduled' to occur each week at first and then at more widely spaced intervals.

(5) The contract provides a simple record of how much reinforcement or punishment is received by each side. The format of the contract also makes it clear how much reinforcement is possible, when it can be obtained and the conditions which would cancel its availability.

Contingency contracting has been used widely with problem drinkers,[14] delinquents in residential settings[15] and at home[16] with schoolchildren[17] and with psychiatric patients[18].

Reciprocity Counselling. A special kind of contract has been developed for use with couples experiencing marital discord.[19] In reciprocity counselling both husband and wife collaborate with the therapist in shaping their relationship to their mutual satisfaction. The package lists ten aspects of the marital relationship. Both partners are encouraged to assess the 'contributions' made by their spouse, rating how 'happy' or 'unhappy' they are with each of the factors — e.g. 'household responsibilities', 'bringing up the children', 'money', 'sex', etc. Both partners identify what they do which pleases their partner and what the partner does in turn, on each factor. Finally, they identify a new contribution which, if their partner would agree to do this, would make them very happy. The ratings, and perceived giving and receiving of 'pleasures', provide an objective basis for discussing the assets and deficits of the relationship. The contract, which is often only verbal, involves both partners in reciprocal *positive* reinforcement. This allows each partner to control the other by positive means, rather than by punishment tactics.

Modelling

Much of our behaviour is learned vicariously, by observing and imitating other people's behaviour. Children model themselves initially upon their parents and later upon members of their peer group. When we grow up we may continue to model ourselves upon our respective cultural or social peer groups or upon 'high status' models such as authority figures or fashionable stars of films or television, etc. Although modelling is more complex than simple 'mimicry' (see Chapter 2), it does rely upon the collaboration of nurse and patient in the performance of the same behaviour. The technique has three major applications: establishing basic skills, weakening avoidance behaviour and increasing the performance of existing behaviour patterns.

Characteristics of the Model.   Bandura[20] suggests that the model should be able to hold the patient's attention, to gain his trust, be a realistic reference figure and be able to demonstrate plausible standards of behaviour for the patient concerned. Although the model does not have to be the same age, sex and cultural background as the patient, in some cases this may be helpful. Bandura emphasises that the model should be *relevant* and *credible*.

Building Basic Social Skills.   Lovaas and his colleagues[21] used modelling in the establishment of basic skills in autistic children. The early goals of the programme involved teaching the child to imitate non-verbal behaviour and to use this imitative ability to promote other social behaviours. Initially an adult modelled the behaviour — e.g. picking up and placing a ball or block — and then prompted the unresponsive child to imitate his actions. As the programme progressed these prompts were faded as the child began to imitate the actions more readily. From this simple beginning Lovaas proceeded to establish other social or pro-social skills: using the toilet, playing, rule-following, smiling and nodding during social interaction. Modelling played a large part in establishing these behaviour patterns and was also used in the final phase of the programme where imitative and then functional speech was established. At this level, modelling operates as another prompting technique, 'cueing' the child to perform the target behaviour which will then be reinforced. This technique plays a large part in treatment and training programmes with the mentally handicapped and other people with skill deficit problems.

Weakening Avoidance Behaviour. Modelling can also be used to reduce fears, which are expressed by avoidance of animals, heights, crowds, etc. One of the most effective ways of treating such phobic reactions is by *participant modelling*. After watching the model interact *safely* with the feared situation, patient and model perform the 'approach' behaviour together. In some cases a hierarchy would be used, beginning with the least threatening and working up gradually to the most feared situation. At each stage the patient is praised and given further encouragment, as he imitates the model's behaviour. As treatment progresses the amount of modelling and additional instruction is reduced, allowing the patient to face the feared situation independently. Bandura emphasises that mere exposure to the feared situation is not enough: the session should be controlled to ensure that the patient can imitate the model safely and successfully. This is especially important in the early stages of treatment. If a dog-phobic is accidentally bitten by a 'snappy' dog, or a crowd-phobic is jostled by a teenage gang, this may reinforce their fear and increase their avoidance behaviour.

In a classic experiment Bandura described the use of participant modelling with snake-phobics.[22] Initially the patients watched the model through a one-way mirror as he picked up and handled the smake. During a 15-minute period he held the snake close to his face and allowed it to slither over his body. After returning it to the cage the patients were brought into the room and seated near to the snake cage. The model then went through increasingly fear-evoking stages of contact with the snake. He asked the patients to imitate his actions of touching, then stroking and finally holding the snake, at first with gloved and then with bare hands. If any patient was unwilling to do this, he was asked to touch the model's hand as he contacted the snake and to move his own hand gradually towards the snake.

Social Skills Training. Although social skills deficits are not peculiar to psychiatric or mentally handicapped patients, inept or embarrassing social behaviour can severely restrain the life-style of such patients. The patient may be unable to 'read' cues or signals given during conversation; others may find him irritating or a 'wet blanket' as a result. Often the patient will complain of not knowing what to say or do when in company. This 'awkward' or 'embarrassing' style may be accompanied by anxiety, where the patient is aware of his difficulties. Otherwise the patient may be confused as to why he 'cannot get along with other people'. Social skills training uses modelling to teach subtle patterns of non-verbal behaviour, upon which 'communication' is based and to demonstrate the kind of verbal content which is appropriate to different kinds of social encounter. Specific packages have been developed for acute[23] and chronic[24] psychiatric patients and the mentally handicapped. An illustration of modelling within an assertion training group is given in Chapter 9.

Exposure Methods

One of the major features of situation-specific anxiety is the avoidance of the feared object or setting. This avoidance pattern may disrupt the patient's lifestyle, each day being devoted to ensuring that the patient does not come within range of the fear-evoking situation. Exposure techniques involve reversing this avoidance pattern of behaviour and encouraging the patient to *approach* the feared situation.

Graded Exposure. Where the patient is extremely afraid of a situation he can be helped to approach this gradually, taking it 'one step at a time'. Using a hierarchy (see Chapter 8), the patient is encouraged at first to face the least-feared situation, progressing gradually through defined stages until he can face the most threatening situation. Repeated *successful* exposure extinguishes the fear reaction: the catastrophe which the patient expects, never materialises. Graded exposure, combined with modelling, is a valuable approach, particularly with the mentally handicapped and other severely disabled people who may not benefit from the anxiety management methods described in Chapter 8.

Flooding. In flooding, or prolonged exposure, the patient is not introduced to the feared situation gradually, but is 'put in at the deep end'. He is asked to spend long periods — often up to two hours — in the situation which evokes *most* anxiety.[25] Few patients select this approach if alternatives are available. However, where there are limitations on therapy time, as in exam or travel phobias, it may be necessary to treat the avoidance behaviour quickly. Before the session begins the patient is given an explanation of what is about to happen, how long the session will last, how he will feel at first (high anxiety) and how this is likely to taper off as the session progresses (extinction). Advice about relaxation may be given and modelling plus social reinforcement provided throughout the flooding session; once again this will be faded gradually over the sessions. It is important to ensure that the patient does not have any means of escape from the session, as this will negatively reinforce the fear reaction. Homework assignments are given to maintain the patient's exposure in everyday life, as a supplement to formal therapy sessions.

Self-treatment Methods

Where the patient is motivated to overcome his problems of living and is capable of controlling his behaviour, he may be able to use many of the techniques already described, in a self-treatment programme. In this situation the nurse's role is to plan assignments, to teach the use of specific techniques and to monitor the patient's progress from his self-observation records. Although self-control has long been seen as a function of 'willpower' or 'ego-strength', behavioural self-control is something a person *does* rather than something which he *has*. Self-control techniques can be divided into five major categories: stimulus control, self-monitoring, self-reward or self-punishment, alternate response training and cognitive methods. (The cognitive self-control techniques involve change 'from within' and are discussed in the next chapter.)

Stimulus Control

Many behaviour patterns are under the control of environmental 'cues'. Traffic lights 'cue' both driver and pedestrian behaviour; a church cues whispering, whereas a sports ground cues shouting. Certain behaviours occur in the presence of specific discriminative stimuli because we have been taught to respond in this way to these cues, or because associations between our behaviour and these cues have developed accidentally. For instance, if we always eat our meals while watching television, the sight of the television may become a discriminative stimulus for eating and we may feel hungry.

In stimulus control the patient is taught to recognise the factors which cue certain patterns of behaviour. An overweight person would be taught to recognise and control the situations which normally encourage him to eat or an insomniac to recognise the situations which cue him to stay awake, such as reading in bed. Goldiamond[26] described a patient who was told that he could 'eat to his heart's content', provided that he always set the table completely, even for a biscuit. He was also told that while eating he must not engage in any other behaviour, such as reading or watching television. The patient may also be told how to reduce the likelihood of engaging in certain behaviours, by controlling his access to materials which are needed to carry out the behaviour. Smokers might leave their cigarettes at home; a 'spend-thrift' might leave his cheque book at home when he went shopping. Stimulus control methods have been used successfully to reduce habitual behaviours, such as eating and smoking, and also to overcome studying problems and insomnia.[27]

Self-monitoring

As we discussed in Chapter 6 the simple act of observing our own behaviour can produce a *reactivity* effect, leading to increases or decreases in behaviour. Although it is not clear why this should happen, several studies involving a wide range of patient populations have documented this effect.[28,29] Where the patient is worried about his behaviour, as in overeating or smoking, recording each mouthful eaten or cigarette smoked may act like a form of punishment. Where the behaviour is part of a sequence of actions, noting down what has just been done may break up the chain of behaviours. Patients may be asked to monitor both sides of a problem. A smoker might record each cigarette smoked, but may also monitor the number of times he refused a cigarette. Self-monitoring is likely to increase the frequency of behaviour which the patient evaluates 'positively' − such as refusing a cigarette − and to decrease 'negatively evaluated' behaviours. Research suggests that the effects of self-monitoring are likely to be short-lived; in this sense it is very similar to observer effect. For this reason the patient should add self-praise to the monitoring exercise, to reinforce the reactivity effect.

Self-reward and Self-punishment

Patients can use reinforcement and punishment techniques to control their behaviour in a 'personal contract'. Although this may be purely 'verbal', a formal written agreement, between the patient and *himself*, witnessed by the nurse, may be helpful in some cases. Rewards or punishments can be 'self-administered' under the nurse's supervision. Overweight patients, who have paid money into a 'kitty' at the start of treatment, can reward or punish themselves with receipt or forfeiture of specific sums of money, as they achieve or fail at weight loss targets. A college student, who was very active in a political party, 'contracted' to forfeit money to a rival political party, if he failed to complete homework or to carry out his socialisation assignments. The student brought any 'forfeited' money with him to the clinic each week and was required to address and mail this in the presence of the therapist.

Most self-reward or punishment strategies use the Premack Principle: the patient only allows himself access to high probability behaviours — such as going to the cinema or seeing a friend — if he has achieved certain specified targets. Alternatively he requires himself to engage in low probability behaviour, such as extra work or complimenting a sworn enemy, if he fails to meet that goal.

The role of models in the patient's learning history plays a part in determining how he will use reward and punishment. Some patients find it easy to punish themselves and need to be coaxed into acknowledging their 'successes', whereas for other patients the reverse is the case. Bandura suggests that this is a function of vicarious learning (see Chapter 2). Patients tend to model themselves upon self-reinforcing *or* self-punishing stereotypes. The nurse can use modelling to good effect, to encourage patients to be more rewarding or more critical with themselves, whichever is appropriate.

Alternate Response Training

Self-relaxation. Many patients experience excessive tension or anxiety and can be taught how to relax and to bring the anxiety under some control. Self-relaxation is based upon the early work of Jacobsen in the 1930s. The patient is taught how to relax the major muscle groups of his body, beginning with the arms, then legs, trunk, back and finally head and neck. The first session may take 20–30 minutes, after which the patient is instructed to carry out the self-relaxation at home, often with the assistance of tape-recorded instructions (see Appendix 5). By alternately tensing and relaxing different muscle groups the patient learns to discriminate the feelings of tension and relaxation. Whenever he begins to feel tense, or is preparing for a stressful encounter, he practises self-relaxation.

Habit Reversal. Where the patient is engaging in some 'automatic' behaviour — such as tics, hair-pulling or nail-biting — he is taught to detect the *beginning* of this behaviour, after which he practises an isometric exercise which is incompatible with the problem behaviour. This usually takes the form of tensing of the muscles of the arm or fist, for about two minutes, following detection of hair-pulling, nail-biting, etc. The same procedure is used when the patient has an 'urge' to perform the behaviour.

A variant of this technique involves the patient in a gradual reduction of the problem behaviour. A woman who repeatedly scratched itchy rashes on her legs was told to stroke her legs whenever she felt like scratching them. This was later converted to patting. At each stage the alternative response helped reduce the target scratching behaviour.[30],[31]

Summary

In this chapter we have discussed the techniques which can change behaviour 'from the outside'. These methods, all of which involve making changes in the environmental conditions which 'stimulate' or 'maintain' the problem behaviour, can be classed under three main headings:

(1) Those methods which are controlled by a 'therapist'. A specially trained 'behaviour therapist', nurses on a hospital ward, or some 'significant other' such as the patient's parents, selects appropriate treatment goals and 'engineers' the patient towards these targets by careful manipulation of conditions in his environment. Existing behaviour patterns can be increased or decreased by reinforcement or punishment contingencies. Where the desired behaviour is absent, this can be established by use of a range of prompting techniques. Once the patient can show the behaviour ir can be developed by use of reinforcement techniques and strengthened by the use of reinforcement schedules.

(2) Those methods which require the collaboration of patient and therapist. Although the nurse may use many of the prompting and reinforcement methods described above, collaborative methods are characterised by nurse and patient working together. The patient may have the opportunity to negotiate the conditions of therapy, as in contingency contracting. Alternatively, he may learn from experience of the nurse, as she models appropriate social behaviour, or demonstrates how to face a feared-situation. Where problems have to be treated quickly, at great emotional cost to the patient, the nurse again provides modelling and 'moral' support.

(3) Those methods which the patient can use to treat himself, through a self-control programme. The nurse's role in self-directed programmes is to teach the use of specific techniques and to provide

additional reinforcement for progress, when nurse and patient meet to discuss the programme. Where the patient's motivation is limited, a contract can be built into the programme.

The treatment methods described in this chapter are applicable to a wide range of problems and, since they are reliant only upon 'external' factors, can be applied to a wide cross-section of patients. Some of these approaches are taken a stage further in Chapter 8, which deals with change from 'within'. A number of illustrations of external control techniques are given in Chapter 9.

Notes

1. Skinner, B.F. *Beyond Freedom and Dignity* (Harmondsworth, Penguin Books, 1973), pp. 91–2.

2. For a scale developed for out-patients, see: Cautela, J.R. 'Reinforcement survey schedule: evaluation and current applications', *Psychological Reports*, vol. 30 (1972), pp. 683–90.

3. For a scale developed for in-patients, see: Cautela, J.R. and Kastenbaum, R. 'A reinforcement survey schedule for use in therapy, training and research', *Psychological Reports*, vol. 20 (1967), pp. 1115–30.

4. For a comprehensive review of research, see: Kazdin, A.E. *The Token Economy* (New York, Plenum Press, 1977).

5. For a detailed description of the use of prompting and fading, along with other operant techniques, see: Watson, L.S. *How to Use Behaviour Modification with Mentally Retarded and Autistic Children* (Columbus, Ohio, Behaviour Modification Technology, 1972).

6. Isaacs, W., Thomas, J. and Goldiamond, I. 'Application of operant conditioning to reinstate verbal behaviour in psychotics', *Journal of Speech and Hearing Disorders*, vol. 25 (1960), pp. 8–12.

7. For an example of backward chaining used in dressing, see: Moore, P. and Carr, J. 'Behaviour modification programme', *Nursing Times* (2 September 1976), pp. 1356–9. See also Chapter 9.

8. Whitman, T.L., Caponigri, V. and Mercurio, J. 'Reducing hyperactive behaviour in a severely retarded child', *Mental Retardation*, vol. 9 (1971), pp. 17–19.

9. Risley, T.R. and Wolf, M.M. 'Establishing functional speech in echolalic children', *Behaviour Research and Therapy*, vol. 5 (1967), pp. 73–88.

10. Sherman, J.A. 'Use of reinforcement and imitation to reinstate verbal behaviour in a mute psychotic', *Journal of Abnormal Psychology*, vol. 70 (1965), pp. 155–64.

11. For a comprehensive review, see: Rachman, S. and Teasdale, J. *Aversion Therapy and Behaviour Disorders: An Analysis* (Coral Gables, Florida, University of Miami Press, 1969).

12. See: Wisley, D.L. and Tough, J. 'Treatment of a self-injuring mongoloid with shock induced suppression and avoidance'. In: R. Ulrich, T. Stachnik and J. Mabry (eds), *Control of Human Behaviour, Vol. 2* (Glenview, Illinois, Scott Foresman, 1970).

13. Ayllon, T. 'Intensive treatment of psychotic behaviour by stimulus satiation and food reinforcement', *Behaviour Research and Therapy*, vol. 1 (1963), pp. 53–62.

14. Miller, P.M. *Behavioural Treatment of Alcoholism* (New York, Pergamon, 1976).

15. Stuart, R.B. and Lott, L.A. 'Behavioural contracting with delinquents: a cautionary note', *Journal of Behaviour Therapy and Experimental Psychiatry*, vol. 2 (1969), pp. 85–92.

16. Weathers, L. and Liberman, R.P. 'Contingency contracting with families of delinquent adolescents', *Behaviour Therapy*, vol. 6 (1975), pp. 356–66.

17. Homme, L.E. *How to Use Contingency Contracting in the Classroom* (Champaign, Illinois, Research Press, 1971).

18. Liberman, R.P. 'Community mental health and behaviour modification: a skeleton in search of muscles that work'. Paper presented at Conference on Community Psychology in Theory and Practice, Western Psychological Association, San Francisco, April 1971.

19. Azrin, N.H. and Naster, B.J. 'Reciprocity counselling: a rapid learning-based procedure for marital counselling', *Behaviour Research and Therapy*, vol. 11 (1973), pp. 365–82.

20. Bandura, A. 'Psychotherapy based upon modeling principles' In: A.E. Bergin and S.L. Garfield (eds), *Handbook of Psychotherapy and Behaviour Change: An Empirical Analysis* (New York, Wiley, 1971).

21. Lovaas, O.I., Frietag, L., Nelson, K. and Whalen, C. 'The establishment of imitation and its use for the development of complex behaviour in schizophrenic children', *Behaviour Research and Therapy*, vol. 5 (1967), pp. 171–81.

22. Bandura, A., Blanchard, E.B. and Ritter, B. 'The relative efficacy of desensitisation and modeling approaches for inducing behavioural, affective and attitudinal changes', *Journal of Personality and Social Psychology*, vol. 13 (1969), pp. 173–99.

23. Trower, P., Bryant, B. and Argyle, M. *Social Skills and Mental Health* (London, Methuen, 1978).

24. Goldstein, A.P., Sprafkin, R.P. and Gershaw, N.J. *Skill Training for Community Living: Applying Structured Learning Therapy* (New York, Pergamon Press, 1976).

25. Marks, I.M., Viswanathan, R. and Lipsedge, M.S. 'Enhanced relief of phobias by flooding during waning effects of diazapam', *British Journal of Psychiatry*, vol. 113 (1967), pp. 711–29.

26. Goldiamond, I. 'Self-control procedures in personal behaviour problems', *Psychological Reports*, vol. 17 (1965), pp. 851–68.

27. For an overview of stimulus control in relation to self-management in general, see: Thoresen, C.E. and Mahoney, M.J. *Behavioural Self-control* (New York, Holt, Rinehart & Winston, 1974), Chapter 1, pp. 17–21.

28. Kanfer, F.H. 'Self-regulation: research issues and speculations'. In: C. Neuringer and J.L. Michael (eds) *Behaviour Modification in Clinical Psychology* (New York, Appleton Century Crofts, 1970).

29. Zegiob, L. 'Reactivity of self-monitoring procedures with retarded adolescents', *American Journal of Mental Deficiency*, vol. 83, no. 2 (1978), pp. 156–63.

30. Watson, D.L., Tharp, R.G. and Krisberg, J. 'Case study in self-modification: suppression of inflammatory scratching while awake and asleep', *Journal of Behaviour Therapy and Experimental Psychiatry*, vol. 3 (1972), pp. 213–15.

31. For a description of habit reversal, see: Rosenbaum, M.S. and Ayllon, T. 'The habit-reversal technique in treating trichotillomania', *Behaviour Therapy*, vol. 12 (1981), pp. 473–81.

8 CHANGING BEHAVIOUR FROM THE INSIDE

> Whether relevant or irrelevant, the things people say
> to themselves determine the rest of the things they do.
> — I.E. Farber

In the last chapter we discussed how behaviour can be changed by manipulating the patient's relationship with his 'outside world'. Problems which inhabit the patient's head may not respond to such methods of control. The patient who experiences obsessional ruminations, thinks about committing suicide, or is hearing 'voices', has a very private problem. Problems may also be mediated by thoughts or fantasies. Anxiety can be aggravated by things people say to themselves. In Chapter 4 we discussed Mrs Smith's self-defeating thoughts: 'things are terrible . . . I'll never get over this . . . I must get out of here'. Although anxiety has certain visible elements — the patient may appear tense or may be running away from a feared situation — the problem also has a hidden element, the internal dialogue between the patient and herself. To solve such a problem successfully on the outside, it may be necessary to change behaviour on the inside.

In a similar vein, a mentally handicapped person who is learning a complex behaviour — such as dressing, laying the table or planning a daily routine — may run into problems if he loses his way along the chain. People often use a 'talk-through' procedure when performing complex actions, especially stressful ones. The person instructs himself, in much the same way as someone would who was showing him how to complete the behaviour. Patients who fail to complete complex chains of behaviour when under stress, or who are erratic in their performance, may need to learn simple 'problem solving' skills to alter their outward show of behaviour.

The Covert and Cognitive Therapies

The techniques discussed in this chapter are aimed at changing covert behaviour — such as obsessional thoughts or auditory hallucinations — or at changing overt behaviour through the use of thinking, imagination or fantasy, in the treatment programme. The techniques described in the last chapter rely to a large extent on therapist control or some outside interference; these methods have a widespread application to a range of patient groups. The covert and cognitive techniques rely more upon collaboration and self-control, and have been used with a more limited range of patients and problems. This does not mean that these methods are applicable only to one patient group. Although acute psychiatric patients are treated most often with these methods, some patients, who have inadequate control over their thinking or imagination etc., may fail to respond. Alternatively, some selected patients from mentally handicapped or chronic psychiatric populations, may respond to a carefully tailored 'covert' treatment plan. The golden rule is to select the treatment method to suit the patient *and* his problem, rather than to prescribe therapy for a particular diagnostic type.

Covert conditioning is part of traditional behaviour therapy, whereas the cognitive therapies are of more recent origin and are the product of a wider range of psychological theories. Cognitive approaches appear to bridge the gulf between radical behaviourism and traditional psychotherapy and are often criticised by the 'radical' school for their investigation of beliefs and values, as part of the therapeutic process. In this chapter I shall discuss the covert techniques which are supported by research evidence and shall discuss the cognitive therapies as an exciting development which may lead to a more comprehensive therapeutic model for a wide variety of patients.

The Covert Techniques

Systematic Desensitisation

Systematic desensitisation (SD) is usually described as a counter-conditioning technique. A stimulus, which normally produces a specific response, is modified by association with a stimulus which produces an incompatible response. SD is used most often to decrease avoidance behaviour, such as phobias. The technique was developed by Joseph Wolpe[1] and involves asking the patient to imagine a series of fear-evoking situations. These are drawn from a *hierarchy*, each stage of which contains a scene which is more anxiety-evoking that the previous one. By 'counter-conditioning', the patient's response to each stage on the hierarchy is changed, producing a reduction in his fear and avoidance.

The technique is based upon the principle that the patient cannot be anxious *and* relaxed at the same time. Wolpe called this *reciprocal inhibition*. He argued that the relationship between the anxiety-evoking stimulus and the anxious response would be weakened if the patient could show 'anxiety-inhibiting' behaviour, when he would normally be anxious. To generate this reciprocal inhibition, Wolpe trained his patients to relax in situations where they would normally be tense.

Systematic desensitisation has three main ingredients:

(1) a graduated hierarchy of anxiety-evoking stimuli;
(2) training in relaxation;
(3) pairing of items on the hierarchy with the relaxed state.

Treatment usually begins with a pre-desensitisation period, when the patient is taught self-relaxation (see Chapter 7). At the same time a hierarchy of feared — or avoided — situations is constructed.

Hierarchy Construction.   The nurse first identifies the anxiety-evoking situations at the initial interview. If the patient has a specific fear, of insects or heights, etc., the hierarchy might describe 'nearness' to the object of his fears: e.g. 'in the same room as a bee' (low anxiety), 'within a foot of a bee' (moderate anxiety), 'with a bee on my arm' (high anxiety). Alternatively, the degree of anxiety might increase by the number of bees, or people, or cars, etc., which are present. In other cases the anxiety may have *generalised* and may be attached to situations only remotely connected with the original fear-stimulus. A young woman who had a fear of people vomiting also experienced anxiety when seeing a dentist's sign, medical advertisements or even drugs, since they were all related in some way to 'ill health'. In extreme cases of generalised phobias the patient may avoid a number of situations which appear unconnected. In such cases it may be helpful to devise several different hierarchies.

The nurse asks the patient to rate each stage on the hierarchy, using a scale from 0 to 100 to record his *subjective units of distress* (suds). Wolpe suggests that 20-25 items should be used, so that only a few points separate one item from the next. However, a ten-stage hierarchy may suffice; additional stages may be added as required during treatment. The patient may be asked to list his fear-situations, as a homework assignment. These will provide the framework for the hierarchy construction at the next session.

The Desensitisation Session.   After the patient has mastered the relaxation — which may take up to two weeks of twice-daily practice — the desensitisation begins. The dialogue between the nurse and the patient with the vomit-phobia went as follows:

Nurse: Have you been practising your relaxation exercise?
Patient: Yes. I'm doing them for about twenty minutes, twice a day. But I'm sure that the relaxed feeling isn't spreading. I mean, I'm just as frightened and tense as ever.
Nurse: Well we're going to look at that today. Can you just lie back in the chair . . . that's fine, just relax and stretch out . . . take a minute or two . . . when you feel nice and relaxed raise the fore-finger of your right hand. (patient signals) OK how much anxiety are you feeling just now?
Patient: None at all.
Nurse: Right. Now I'd like you to imagine that you are watching TV at home. Your daughter is playing in the next room. Your hus-band is sitting beside you on the couch. Just raise your finger when that picture becomes clear in your mind. (patient signals) Can you tell what you were imagining just then?
Patient: Well. I was sitting at home, like you said. We were watching a film with Paul Newman. My husband and I both like him. Sara was playing with her dolls in the next room. I could hear her talking.
Nurse: Fine. Now just close your eyes again and relax.

The first phase of the session has been used to ensure that the patient can visualise the scene. If she could not, there would be little point in continuing. The nurse asks the patient to relax again: this time she will imagine the first scene on the hierarchy, which evokes a small degree of anxiety. The nurse describes the scene briefly, pausing between descriptions to allow the patient to add her own details. The patient communicates by raising her finger only. This prevents disturbance of the relaxed state. The only time the patient speaks is when giving the *suds* ratings.

Nurse: Imagine that you are sitting at home watching TV. Your daughter comes into the room crying . . . (pause) Your husband asks her what is wrong. Sara says that she doesn't feel well. (pause) When you can visualise that scene raise your finger. (patient signals) Just carry on imagining that scene at home (pause) OK stop imagining the scene now. Raise your finger if you felt any anxiety. (patient signals) How much did you feel?

Patient: Oh, about fifteen, I think.

Nurse: Just relax again. Signal when you're fully relaxed. (patient signals) Now imagine that your daughter is coming into the room. She is crying. Your husband asks her what's wrong. She isn't feeling well. Signal when you have pictured it. (patient signals) Now carry on imagining that scene at home. (pause) OK stop there. Did you feel any anxiety?

Patient: Well not so much that time. About ten. Maybe less.

Nurse: OK. Just let yourself relax. Signal when you're ready.

The nurse continues repeating the scene until the patient experiences no anxiety. She would then move on to the next stage in the hierarchy, repeating the relaxation and imagination process. If the suds rating does not reduce after repeated presentation, the scene is presented in a milder form or for a shorter period. This session lasts for about twenty minutes: the nurse cues the patient to relax and imagine the scene on the hierarchy, moving on as the anxiety extinguishes. At the end of the session the nurse negotiates a homework assignment which will allow the patient to face a real-life situation which is similar to the one dealt with in imagination during the session. An agoraphobic might be asked to cross the street from her house to post a letter, or a height-phobic might look out of the upstairs bedroom window when it is closed. In the case illustrated above the patient was asked to put her daughter to bed each night and to give her her cough medicine. The patient is advised about the use of relaxation during the exposure assignment. At the next session the patient reports back on the 'homework' and discusses ways of overcoming any practical difficulties. The next desensitisation session begins at the stage on the hierarchy which was completed successfully at the last session.

Practical Problems.   Some patients may find it difficult to relax, especially if they are embarrassed by the nurse watching them. This can be overcome by sitting slightly to the rear of the patient. The patient may also be given a prerecorded tape of the nurse reading the instruction. If he is given an opportunity to practise alone and free from distraction, this may expedite relaxation within the session.

Other patients may have difficulty imagining the scene, may be distracted by intrusive thoughts or may not become anxious when imagining the scenes. For these patients graded exposure might be a more appropriate treatment. In other cases the patient may fail to habituate to a particular scene on the hierarchy. Two solutions are possible. The patient may continue imagining the scene until habituation takes place or an additional item can be added to the hierarchy, spanning the one where he has 'stuck' and the last item completed successfully.

Applications and Comments. Systematic desensitisation has been used for specific phobias, (e.g. for heights, darkness, animals, etc.), social anxieties (where it may be used as an adjunct to assertion training – see Chapter 9) and sexual dysfunction. Although the approach has been successful,[2] there is still much argument about *why* it works. Although Wolpe's model is based upon relaxation, this is not always an essential ingredient. Some authors stress the importance of covert behaviours involved. In a classic study with public-speaking phobics Paul[3] asked his subjects to imagine themselves *in* the feared situation, rather than simply observing it as in a film. Although evidence to support the importance of these symbolic events is lacking, the imaginal *experience* of the situation may be an important ingredient. Mahoney[4] suggests that the patient should be asked to feel himself in the situation, hearing sounds and feeling sensations – such as the contours of a seat or smells – which are appropriate. This strategy may also overcome the problem of unresponsiveness. Mahoney has also pointed out that positive imagery can be an effective 'inhibiting' agent. In a study with pepticulcer patients[5] an experimental group reported a greater degree of symptomatic relief when they imagined pleasant scenes, whenever they felt anxious. The use of positive imagery, in a fantasy scene, was used by Lazarus and Abramovitz,[6] in treating a ten-year-old boy. The therapist paired anxiety with scenes involving comic book heroes:

Now I want you to close your eyes and imagine that you are sitting in the dining room with your father and mother. It is night time. Suddenly you receive a signal on your wrist radio that Superman gave you. You quickly run into the lounge because your mission must be kept secret. There is only a little light coming into the lounge from the passage. Now pretend that you are all alone in the lounge waiting for Superman and Captain Silver to visit you.

This example emphasises the use of imagery which is carefully scripted to suit the child. Mahoney argues that *appropriate* imagery, in terms of a realistic description of the scene, and positive covert behaviour, where the patient thinks pleasing, exciting or stimulating thoughts, are more relevant to the counter-conditioning process. This is especially so in situations where relaxation might be an inappropriate response. Although there has been little use of systematic desensitisation with the mentally handicapped, the example above shows how the process can be adapted to suit the individual patient.

Thought-stopping

Although popularised by Wolpe, thought-stopping was first used in the late twenties. The procedure is used most often to reduce obssessional ruminations, but has also been described as a way of reducing auditory and visual hallucinations. The patient engages in the troublesome thoughts and the therapist interrupts him by shouting 'Stop' loudly. This may be accompanied by banging the table, clapping hands or giving the patient a mild electric shock. This startles him and terminates the thoughts for a few minutes. The effect of this distraction is pointed out to the patient and the process repeated. This time the patient shouts 'Stop' as soon as he engages in the unwanted thoughts. This is repeated several times until he can interrupt the thoughts by saying 'Stop' *to himself.*

The Procedure. A young man who suffered from severe social anxiety described a number of self-defeating thoughts: 'who wants to talk to a fool like me . . . I'm so ugly no one listens to me . . .' The dialogue between nurse and patient went as follows:

Nurse: I want you to imagine that you are going into the lounge bar at your local. It is a cold dark evening . . . the lights are bright as you step inside. Close your eyes and picture the scene. A group of people are standing at the bar, with their backs to you. One of the girls turns as you come in and smiles. As you think about the scene thoughts will pop into your head. I want you to say aloud what you are thinking about this situation.

Patient: (Pauses for a few seconds) I'm wondering why I came in here. I'd like to order a drink but I'm a bit embarrassed. They're probably talking about how I look. Laughing at me. They're probably saying I look . . .

Nurse: (Shouting) STOP! (pause for a few seconds) That was designed to break your pattern of thinking. Can you tell me what happened?

Patient: Well I got a shock. I didn't expect it.

Nurse: Did it interfere with your thinking?

Patient: Well, yes. I just wondered 'what's up?'

Nurse: OK. Let's try it again. Imagine the scene and tell me what you are thinking.

The nurse repeats the exercise, shouting 'Stop' as soon as the patient articulates some self-defeating thoughts. At the same time he is encouraged to think 'positively': each time he speaks a positive thought aloud the nurse reinforces this — 'Uh huh, very good, etc.' Once the thoughts are being 'stopped' consistently, the nurse proceeds to stop covert thoughts, interrupting the patient as before whenever he signals that he is engaging in a self-defeating thought. The patient is then asked to shout 'Stop' himself. Usually patients are reticent at first, but the nurse can model more emphatic 'stopping' or can 'shape' this by gradual encouragement.

Once the patient can stop his thoughts in this manner the nurse explains the need to establish a *covert* stopping tactic:

> *Nurse:* Now it's obvious that you can't go around shouting 'Stop' whenever you're troubled by negative thoughts. People really would start looking at you. (patient laughs) Let's see if you can stop these thoughts by saying 'Stop' under your breath. Perhaps if you move your tongue and feel the tightening in your throat as you 'say' it that will help.
>
> *Patient:* Should I close my eyes again?
>
> *Nurse:* If you like. The important thing is to picture the scene and to let the thoughts come and then really shout out that 'Stop'. Only this time don't shout. Keep the whole effect on the inside.

The nurse encourages the patient to practise this several times. Once he has learned to block these thoughts a homework assignment is set up to give him a chance to practise in the situation where they are most prevalent. Thought-stopping is a simple technique for blocking out unwanted thoughts, but, in addition, the nurse should be encouraging appropriate thoughts, as she discusses the patient's view of difficult situations. There may also be some value in introducing humour, to lighten what may be a grim session.

Overview of the Procedure. Thought-stopping can be summarised in the following stages:

(1) The nurse discusses the patient's negative thoughts, trying to persuade him of their self-defeating nature.
(2) The patient is asked to speak these thoughts aloud as he imagines the problem situation. The nurse then interrupts the beginning of the thought pattern by shouting 'Stop'.

(3) The patient signals when he is thinking unwanted thoughts and the nurse repeats the 'Stop' procedure.
(4) The patient 'Stops' himself whenever the thoughts occur.
(5) The patient uses a covert 'stopping' tactic when thoughts occur.
(6) The patient uses this covert tactic in real-life as a homework assignment.

Rimm[7] adds a further stage to the procedure by encouraging the patient to make an assertive response, following the thought-stopping. Patients are instructed to say something assertive aloud at first; the patient in our illustration might say 'I'm as smart as any other guy here . . . or . . . I like the look of that girl over there'. The patient must create an assertive response which suits him. The nurse should avoid 'feeding' him with an appropriate statement. Once he has practised this aloud, this assertive response is also made covertly.

Applications.   Thought-stopping has been used widely with obsessive ruminations and phobic problems like the one illustrated, where the patient has some self-defeating thoughts. It has also been used to reduce auditory hallucinations[8] and visual hallucinations[9]. Mahoney[10] encouraged a patient to snap a heavy gauge rubber band on his wrist whenever he said 'Stop', adding a tactile aversive element. Case reports show that there are wide variations in the use of the technique. This has made evaluation of the procedure difficult. Although case reports are encouraging, controlled studies[11] have shown disappointing results. This may be due to the way in which the procedure is adapted by individual practitioners. Mahoney has doubts about the reasons why the technique is said to work. He points out that not all ruminations or other covert problems are verbal; in many cases the problem involves imagery, rather than discrete thoughts. However, it is a simple technique which the patient can learn easily and is useful as a preliminary method for controlling distressing thoughts.

Covert Sensitisation

This technique was first described by Cautela[12] as a form of symbolic aversion therapy. The procedure involves giving the patient some relaxation training, then asking him to picture himself in the problem situation. The nurse then relates the 'script' of the scene. The following extract, from the treatment of a patient with an overeating problem, is influenced strongly by Cautela's approach.

I want you to imagine that you are dining with friends. You have just finished your main course and your friend passes you some trifle. As you look at it you feel a little queasy. You pick up the spoon and begin to feel even more nauseous. As you start to spoon the trifle, you feel an acid taste at the back of your throat. As you raise the spoon to your mouth you feel that you are going to be sick. Some food comes up your throat. You cough a little; raising your hand to your mouth to try to hold it back. You feel a slight shudder in your throat as you raise the spoonful of trifle to your mouth. As you are about to open your mouth you are violently sick. The vomit goes all over your plate on to the table, spilling down your best dress. Tears are streaming from your eyes as you vomit again. The vomit splashes on to the person sitting next to you. There is a terrible stench as everyone turns to look at you. Someone offers you a handkerchief, but you vomit again all over him. You turn away from the table and immediately feel better. You run out of the room and into the bathroom. You are feeling better and better. As you wash yourself the terrible feeling leaves you completely and you feel wonderful.

Cautela's approach often involves nausea. This is timed to follow the imagined performance of the maladaptive behaviour, in this case eating trifle. However, any kind of aversive imagery may be used. Case reports often describe shameful experiences, as in the illustration where other people are involved. A 'shame' image was used in the treatment of a man with homosexual tendencies.[13] The patient was instructed to imagine picking up, and becoming sexually involved with a man, only to be caught by his wife. Highly personal aversive imagery can also be used. Kolvin[14] used a 'fear of falling' — which the patient experienced in dreams — in the treatment of a young fetishist.

The finale of the scene always uses some 'relief' sequence: the patient feels better after turning away from the source of his problems. Often a specific 'aversion relief' scene is used, where the patient feels better as a result of restraining his impulse to eat, drink or engage in some deviant sexual behaviour: 'You are about to start eating the trifle when you start to feel sick all over. You think to yourself . . . "I'm not going to eat that trifle . . . I'm trying to lose weight anyway." As soon as you say this you feel quite relaxed and the nauseous feeling passes.'

Applications. The success of covert sensitisation varies according to the problem treated. It has had little effect on smoking and drinking, faring only slightly better with overeating. The approach has been most successful with sexual deviations. Mahoney suggests that this may be because these typically involve fantasies and erotic *imagery*, whereas smoking, drinking and eating are more 'automatic', with little in the way of mediating influences. However the technique is unlikely to be harmful and can be offered to the overweight or the problem drinker as another self-control technique, which can be discarded if unsuccessful.

Covert Modelling

This technique is based on Bandura's research into symbolic and participant modelling. The patient visualises someone performing behaviour which is incompatible with his problem. Although early support came from Cautela's case reports, the technique has been studied most closely by Kazdin.[15]

Procedure.   The patient imagines someone in a situation which gives him problems. A dog-phobic might imagine someone walking down a street or in a park, an unassertive patient, someone confronting a shop assistant. The instructions might go as follows:

> I want you to imagine that you are watching someone walking through the park on his way home. He sees a large dog crossing the park towards him. It is an Alsatian and appears to be on its own. He continues walking across the grass and the dog brushes against his legs as he passes it. Although it is a large dog, he does not stop. The dog runs off into the distance.

The kind of scene described above is a 'mastery' model. The person is very competent by comparison with the patient and shows no fear at all. Alternatively, a 'coping' model could be used:

> Imagine that you are watching a man walking through the park. He sees a large dog running across the grass towards him. He hesitates for a moment, slowing his pace a little. The dog stops a few feet away from him and stands looking at him. The man stops and relaxes himself, taking a few deep breaths. He steps forward and walks past the dog which watches him as he passes. The dog then runs off in the opposite direction.

In this example the model is more like the patient, hesitating and showing tension. The model then shows how to cope with the situation, relaxing, taking deep breaths, etc. Kazdin's studies of covert modelling have produced the following conclusions:

(1) A coping model is preferable to a mastery one.
(2) The age and sex of the model should match that of the patient.
(3) Covert reinforcement will enhance the effects of modelling. A positive event — such as the dog walking away, or a shopkeeper apologising, in the description — will increase the likelihood of the patient imitating the model in real life.

Covert modelling has also been used to treat alcoholics and obssessive compulsive behaviour.[16] A novel report involved a child who consistently lit fires with matches.[17] The child was told a story, illustrated with pictures and dolls, about a boy who found matches and gave them to his mother, who said what a clever boy he was, and gave him some sweets. The child was then asked to tell the story to the therapist, including the favourable consequences for 'good behaviour'. At the same time the child's mother was told to praise him and give him a reward, if he ever brought her matches, thereby turning the fantasy into reality.

Summary of Covert Techniques

The four techniques described are covert methods since they rely heavily upon imagination and fantasy, etc. They also depend upon the therapist to design the imaginal sequences and to direct the session. Nurse and patient also collaborate, to ensure that the sequences designed fit the patient's requirements. Although Cautela argues that these techniques are based upon 'recognised learning theories', such as operant and classical conditioning, this view may be an oversimplification. Since these theories do not explain overt behaviour adequately, they cannot be used to explain covert behaviour. Many researchers acknowledge that these methods work, but are uncertain why. This shows that existing theories of human behaviour are inadequate to some extent. The examples given illustrate, however, that covert techniques have much to offer a range of patient populations and problems, providing that they are handled with care and perhaps some creativity.

In recent years more interest has been shown in cognitive or information-processing research. Mahoney has suggested that some of the success of covert techniques may be derived from a cognitive-information model, especially where the patient learns how to rehearse behaviour on a 'mental' level. Although the use of imagery in 'mental practice' is hardly new, it is now being shaped into a number of specific treatment methods which we shall now discuss.

The Cognitive Therapies

Self-instructional Training

Although 'self-talk' has been recognised for centuries as a way of regulating emotions and generating behaviour, it has been studied only recently within behaviour therapy. Self-instruction, as a means for producing patterns of overt behaviour, was first studied by Meichenbaum.[18] His work had added interest since it involved schizophrenics, whom he taught to 'talk healthy'. This led to studies in which psychotic patients learned to control their verbal and social behaviour, by 'talking to themselves'.

Self-instruction has been used as an approach for solving 'impulsive' behaviour in children. Meichenbaum described a process which parallels the way in which normal children internalise their speech:

(1) An adult models the target behaviour — e.g. fitting jigsaw pieces or dressing — while instructing himself aloud.

(2) The child is asked to imitate the adult's behaviour; the adult instructs the child throughout.

(3) The child is then asked to perform the task instructing himself aloud.

(4) The child repeats the task, this time whispering the instructions to himself.

(5) Finally, the child performs the behaviour, guiding his perform-ance by self-instruction ('private speech').

In this procedure the adult provides *cognitive modelling* in stage (1), showing the child how to 'think-through' the behaviour. The action is consolidated in stage (2) under instruction and in (3) and (4) the child internalises the instructions gradually. The self-instruction is established in stage (5). Meichenbaum and Goodman[19] give an example of cogni-tive modelling at the first stage, where the target behaviour is copying a pattern:

OK what is it I have to do? You want me to copy the picture with the different lines. I have to go slow and be careful. OK draw the

line down, down, good; then to the right, that's it; now down some
more and to the left. Good, I'm doing fine so far. Remember, go
slow. Now back up again. No, I was supposed to go down. That's
OK. Just erase the line carefully . . . Good. Even if I make an error I
can go on slowly and carefully. OK. I have to go down. Finished.
I did it.

This illustrates the important elements of self-instructional training.
The model asks himself 'what have I to do?' He focuses his attention
on the required behaviour '. . . be careful. Okay, draw the line down'.
At various points in the sequence the model reinforces himself, 'good,
I'm doing fine'. Finally, he models coping with an error. Although the
example appears simple, it embraces a definition of the target behaviour, performance guidelines, self-reinforcement and a coping
strategy. Since the task is likely to be difficult for the patient, a coping
– rather than a mastery – model is recommended.

Although self-instructional training is similar to many self-help
manuals, there is a world of different between the highly specific and
task-relevant self-statements modelled by Meichenbaum, and 'positive
thinking' books. In self-instructional training the patient learns how to
solve problems, cope with the stress of failure and to promote adaptive
behaviour by self-reinforcement. Although the technique is somewhat
remote from the laboratory experiments of B.F. Skinner, it also
emphasises an analysis of the patient's behavioural difficulties. Although
the method has had only limited application, it can be incorporated
into self-care and play skills training with some mentally handicapped
patients and has a number of possibilities in the psychiatric rehabilita-
ton setting.

Stress Inoculation

This technique is a variant of self-instructional training, and is used in
conjunction with self-relaxation. Although stress inoculation has been
used most widely with phobic reactions, it has been applied, more
recently, to anger and pain control. Stress inoculation has four stages:

(1) Preparing for the stressor: the patient is encouraged to offer
self-statements which will help him prepare for the stressful situation.
He might be facing an audience, entering a supermarket or walking past
a dog. The nurse may need to model appropriate thoughts, but should
always try to shape up the patient's own version. Typical self-statements
might be:

Okay. What have I to do here? Just think about what you need to do. Don't worry, that won't help you at all. Just concentrate on the task in hand. That's right, just think about what you want to do. You're feeling a little anxious. That's only natural. You're probably a little excited. Just get on with it.

(2) Confronting the stressor: the patient is then encouraged to make self-statements which will help him manage his anxiety, once he is in the situation. By now he may have begun his speech, stepped into the shop, or be standing beside the dog. Typical self-statements might be:

You can do it. I know you can! Just take it easy. Keep your mind on what you're doing. That's right. Okay, you're feeling a little wobbly. I never said it would be easy. It'll get better as time passes. Anxiety at this level is only natural. You can handle it anyway. Just relax. Take a deep breath. That's better already!

(3) Coping with panic: the patient rehearses handling extra stress. What will he do if the audience laugh inappropriately, if people start jostling him in the supermarket or if the dog snaps at him? Typical coping statements might be:

If you get frightened just take a breather. Count slowly to ten. Keep your mind on what's next on the list. Don't try to eliminate your fear. That'll just make things worse. Rate your anxiety from 1 to 10. Watch it. See if it's rising or falling.

(4) Reinforcing self-statements: finally the patient is encouraged to reward himself for coping so well. He might say: 'Well done! I knew you could do it. Wait till you tell the others about this. See . . . you made more of the anxiety than you needed to. It's getting better every time you do it.'

Novaco has applied stress inoculation to the control of anger. His 'anger scale'[20] assesses the self-defeating nature of anger, its severity and the provoking situations. The technique has also been used in pain control[21] where a combination of coping self-statements and exposure to pain was more successful than exposure alone.

In the first stage of stress inoculation the nurse discusses the patient's emotional problems, pointing out how they are responses to specific situations. She points out that he may be able to do very little to change these situations. However, between these situations and his emotional reaction, lie certain thoughts. These thoughts determine whether the emotional response is severe or not. To illustrate the power of thought over feelings, the nurse might give an example, viz:

> *Nurse:* As I said, what you say to yourself plays a big part in decid-ing how you feel. Let me give you an example. Imagine that you are alone in the house one night. The house is in darkness: you've just put out all the lights before going to bed. You hear a noise. You think to yourself, 'What's that? Maybe someone is trying to break in.' Now tell me how you would feel.
> *Patient:* Well, pretty terrified, I would think.
> *Nurse:* This time let's imagine that when you hear the noise you say to yourself, 'That'll be that cat I expect, trying to get in the window.' How would you feel?
> *Patient:* Well not frightened. Annoyed perhaps. Maybe angry.

This illustration should demonstrate to the patient how thoughts influence feelings. Most important of all, the patient should learn that feelings do not come 'out of the blue'. The patient is then asked to monitor his thoughts in stress situations, noting down what happens to him, what he thinks about it and how it makes him feel.

The patient is then taught specific coping skills. In addition to the deep relaxation described earlier (see Chapter 7) instruction in cue-controlled relaxation[22] is given, viz:

> Now I want you to become even more relaxed. I want you to study your breathing. Watch how you breathe in . . . and . . . out. Each time you start to breathe out . . . say the word 'relax' to yourself. This word will now become the cue for deeper relaxation.

The patient is then encouraged to volunteer 'personal' coping self-statements, as described earlier. These are used in the preparation, confronting, coping and reinforcing stages of the 'inoculation'. Once the patient has mastered self-statements and relaxation in imagination, the exercise is transferred to real life as a homework assignment.

Cognitive Restructuring

Rational-Emotive Therapy (RET). Although change in thinking patterns is an undercurrent of the techniques already discussed, cognitive restructuring as a specific technique originated in Albert Ellis' 'rational-emotive therapy'. Ellis argued that maladaptive feelings were the product of irrational ideas. He saw these as the root of problems such as depression, anxiety and anger. The following are examples of the kind of irrational ideas which are central to the RET model:

> 'I must be loved by everyone for everything I do.'
> 'Certain actions are awful and wicked and people doing them should be severely punished.'
> 'It is horrible when things are not the way I want them to be.'
> 'My problems are caused by factors outwith my control.'[23]

Since RET has many similarities with Beck's work, which is discussed below, Ellis' approach shall not be discussed further.[24]

Cognitive Therapy (CT). Aaron Beck offers a more organised form of cognitive restructuring, which has become known as 'cognitive therapy'. Beck shares Ellis' view that faulty thinking generates bad feelings. He also rejects the idea of unconscious thought processes popularised by the Freudian movement. Beck argues that the patient must learn to identify and challenge the thoughts which cause his problems. In contrast to Ellis he does not say that these thoughts are always irrational. Instead he suggests that the patient makes *rules* for himself, which are too extreme or absolute and are therefore unworkable. Two main rule-classes can be used to classify self-defeating thoughts:

(1) The *pleasure-pain* class: where the patient believes, for example, that 'I can *never* be happy if I am not famous.'

(2) The *safety-danger* class: where the patient believes, for example, that 'it is *awful* if people criticise me' or 'there is nothing worse than being made to look ridiculous.'

Beck points out that the patient may show his distorted thinking in a number of discrete ways. He may be guilty of:

(1) *Personalisation:* attributing some event, incorrectly, to his own actions — blaming himself for other people's faults.

(2) *Polarised thinking:* seeing events only in 'black-and-white': e.g. things are either right *or* wrong, good *or* bad.

(3) *Selective abstraction:* attending to the details of a situation rather than seeing them in their fuller context.

(4) *Arbitrary inference:* drawing conclusions, usually negative, which are not supported by the facts of the situation.
(5) *Overgeneralisation:* assuming, for example, that he is a total failure, on the basis of a single event.

Overview of Cognitive Therapy. At the beginning of the session the patient is given a simple overview of the treatment model, showing how thinking influences feelings, in the manner described earlier. The patient's problems are then defined and goals set for the treatment programme. In subsequent sessions the format is as follows:

(1) Setting an agenda: the patient is asked what has been 'on his mind' recently. From this are selected the major topics for the session.
(2) Review of the week: the patient is asked to give a brief review of the week and his activities.
(3) Feedback on previous session: the patient is asked to review briefly what happened at the last session.
(4) Review of homework: the patient describes what happened, any problems he met and what he learned from the assignment.
(5) Today's problem: a problem from the agenda is discussed in detail and the core of the session now begins.
(6) Homework assignment: a task is set for the week ahead. An explanation of *why* and *how* the patient should tackle this is given. Difficulties which might arise are discussed and solutions considered.
(7) Feedback: the patient is asked to comment on the session. Are there any points about which he is unclear? Does he have anything to say about the way the session was handled?

Beck favours this structured format since it discourages wasting time in idle chit-chat. He also believes that this structure gives the patient the sense of order which he requires. The maximum number of sessions required for therapy is usually decided at the outset, thereby putting a time-limit on the therapeutic relationship. The cognitive therapy package usually includes a number of behavioural techniques, such as those already described, for use in the early stages of therapy. These are used to demonstrate a relatively simple course of action. Although the core of the cognitive therapy package remains the same, Beck has developed a number of 'approaches' to different problems. In the example below, the CT package is tackling depression. The initial and inter-mediate stages of the treatment involve:

(1) *Activity schedule making:* the patient is encouraged to note down what he is doing from hour to hour each day. He is then encour-aged to engage in simple activities which may elevate his mood, even slightly. With very retarded depressed patients a *graded task* assignment is given: the patient may be encouraged to boil an egg, make up his bed, etc. The tasks are gradually made more difficult, until he is making a complete meal or tidying around the whole house.

(2) *Mastery and pleasure therapy:* the patient is then asked to rate how much satisfaction he gets from performing various tasks. This can be assessed in terms of 'pleasure' – 'how much did he enjoy it?' – or 'mastery' – how much achievement did he feel as a result of doing what he set out to do? Although the patient may get little or no pleasure at first, some mastery ratings will be evident, even if only for simple tasks. These ratings are then used to illustrate that he is not as bad as he once believed.

(3) *Monitoring of automatic thoughts:* as the patient's mood lifts treatment moves on to the cognitive level. The patient is shown how to identify the negative *automatic* thoughts which 'pop into your head'. The patient is asked to keep a record of these thoughts and the feelings which they produce, rating how unpleasant they are and the extent to which he believes 'what is he saying to himself'.

(4) *Challenging automatic thoughts:* once the patient is able to monitor his self-defeating thoughts, he is helped to 'challenge' them in the session. Among the strategies which are used are:

(a) *Disattribution:* helping the patient to recognise that he is not responsible for everything which goes wrong.
(b) *Decatastrophising:* helping the patient to evaluate problems in a more rational manner. In particular he is helped to look at the evidence which supports his view of a particular event.
(c) *Alternative therapy:* helping the patient to work out solutions to what he sees as insoluble problems.

From the very outset the patient's distorted thinking is challenged. This short excerpt from a Beck case report[25] shows how the therapist helps the patient put his problem into perspective.

Client: I have to give a talk before my class tomorrow and I'm scared stiff.

Therapist: What are you afraid of?

Client: I think I'll make a fool of myself.

Therapist: Suppose you do . . . make a fool of yourself. Why is that so bad?

Client: I'll never live it down.

Therapist: 'Never' is a long time . . . Now look here suppose they do ridicule you. Can you die from it?

Client: Of course not.

Therapist: Suppose they decide you're the worst public speaker that ever lived . . . will this ruin your future career?

Client: No . . . but it would be nice if I could be a good speaker.

Therapist: Sure it would be nice. But if you flubbed it, would your parents or your wife disown you?

Client: No . . . they're very sympathetic.

Therapist: Well, what would be so awful about it?

Client: I would feel pretty bad.

Therapist: For how long?

Client: For about a day or two.

Therapist: And then what?

Client: Then I'd be okay.[26]

Simple Cognitive Strategies. Both Beck's and Ellis's approaches are complex to the uninitiated. However, the cognitive therapy of Aaron Beck is likely to become a valuable clinical method because it is well documented, with clear guidelines for the aspiring 'cognitive therapist' from the very first meeting with the patient right through to the end of therapy. Yet it is clear that the essential therapeutic 'style' cannot be picked up overnight and may require a lengthy period of training under supervision. Mahoney suggests that simpler forms of cognitive-change are possible using mnemonic aids to cue the patient to monitor and challenge his self-defeating thoughts. Using the mnemonic ADAPT the patient can analyse difficult situations and can engineer himself towards a more 'adaptive' view of the situation.

Ablett[27] used this mnemonic in a treatment programme with a woman who was diagnosed as manic-depressive psychosis, but who also experienced extreme generalised phobic reactions. Ablett initially modelled appropriate 'approach' behaviour — driving, shopping, socialising — at the same time discussing the patient's thoughts and modelling alternatives. The patient was given modified stress-inoculation and in the third stage of treatment was instructed in the use of the ADAPT mnemonic. The patient wrote out the mnemonic on a cue card which she carried in her handbag, but then memorised. The patient reported a great reduction in her fears and an elevation of mood. After receiving a wide range of treatments over a two-year period, she was most impressed by the 'commonsense' approach offered by Ablett. The ADAPT approach allowed her the opportunity to help herself and showed her that she could bring her problems under her own control.

Summary of the Cognitive Therapies

The cognitive methods described here can be seen as two distinct approaches. Self-instructional training and stress inoculation are very much within the tradition of didactic therapy. The patient is taught how to control his behaviour or how to cope with a specific form of distress; the therapist models and shapes up the desired 'self-statements' in the patient. These two methods hold considerable promise in the treatment of impulsive behaviour or anxiety. They can also be incorporated usefully into treatment programmes as another way of helping the patient establish 'self-control'.

The cognitive restructuring approach of Beck and others is less didactic and much more of a collaborative affair. The therapist is still concerned to help the patient use positive self-statements and to extinguish his self-defeating thoughts. His approach, as the brief extract from the Beck case study shows, is much less direct. Cognitive therapy relies heavily upon the use of Socratic irony: the therapist does not try to persuade the patient that his view of the circumstances is irrational or even wrong. By careful questioning – where he pretends ignorance of the patient's argument – he leads the patient into describing the reality of his situation, by revealing the absurdity of his view of present events: e.g. 'Tell me what would be so bad about that . . . could you die from that?'

Cognitive therapy is the newest departure within behaviour therapy or rather it is the one which has been taken up with great interest by certain behaviour therapists. Both Beck and Ellis come from traditional psychotherapy backgrounds, although they have rejected traditional analytical approaches in favour of their own brands of therapy. The non-behavioural background of cognitive therapy has reinforced the claim that this is not a legitimate area of interest for behaviourists. However, the structure of cognitive therapy and its emphasis upon translating the patient's perception of his problem into discrete 'thoughts', is wholly within the framework of behaviourism, at least as described within this text. It has long been apparent that the things we say to ourselves play a large part in determining our behaviour. It is apparent also that the behaviour of many patients is influenced directly by the way in which they perceive their world. For these patients, the problem is not so much in their environment as in the way they interpret their world. The way we 'see' the outside world can often best be illustrated by the things we say to ourselves about what is happening around us. For many patients our priority may be to help them modify their view of their world and themselves, by helping them change the things they say to themselves.

Notes

1. Wolpe, J. *Psychotherapy by Reciprocal Inhibition* (Stanford, California, Stanford University Press, 1958).

2. See: Bandura, A. *Principles of Behaviour Modification* (New York, Holt, Rinehart & Winston, 1969).

3. Paul, G.L. *Insight versus Desensitisation in Psychotherapy* (Stanford, California, Stanford University Press, 1966).

4. Mahoney, M.J. *Cognition and Behaviour Modification* (Cambridge, Mass., Ballinger, 1974), p. 81.

5. Ibid., pp. 79-80.

6. Lazarus, A.A. and Abramavitz, A. 'The use of "emotive imagery" in the treatment of children's phobias', *Journal of Mental Science*, vol. 108 (1962), pp. 191-5.

7. Rimm, D.C. 'Thought stopping and covert assertion in the treatment of phobias', *Journal of Consulting and Clinical Psychology*, vol. 41 (1973), pp. 466-7.

8. Bucher, B. and Fabricatore, J. 'The use of patient administered shock to suppress hallucinations', *Behaviour Therapy*, vol. 1 (1970), pp. 382-5.

9. Samaan, M. 'Thought stopping and flooding in a case of hallucinations, obssessions and homicidal, suicidal behaviour', *Journal of Behaviour Therapy and Experimental Psychiatry*, vol. 6 (1975), pp. 65-7.

10. Mahoney, *Cognition and Behaviour Modification*, pp. 90-2.

11. Stern, R., Lipsedge, M.S. and Marks, I.M. 'Obsessive ruminations: a controlled trial of thought stopping technique', *Behaviour Research and Therapy*, vol. 11 (1973), pp. 659-62.

12. Cautela, J.R. 'Covert sensitisation for the treatment of sexual deviation', *Psychological Record*, vol. 21 (1971), pp. 37-48.

13. Curtis, R.H. and Presly, A.S. 'The extinction of homosexual behaviour by covert sensitisation: a case study', *Behaviour Research and Therapy*, vol. 10 (1972), pp. 81-3.

14. Kolvin, I. 'Aversion imagery treatment in adolescents', *Behaviour Research and Therapy*, vol. 5 (1967), pp. 245-8.

15. Kazdin, A.E. 'Comparative effects of some variations of covert modeling', *Journal of Behaviour Therapy and Experimental Psychiatry*, vol. 5 (1974), pp. 225-31.

16. Hay, W.M., Hay, L.R. and Nelson, R.O. 'The adaptation of covert modeling procedures to the treatment of chronic alcoholism and obssessive compulsive behaviour: two case reports', *Behaviour Therapy*, vol. 8 (1977), pp. 70-6.

17. Stawar, T.L. 'Fable mod: operantly structured fantasies as an adjunct in the modification of fire setting behaviour', *Journal of Behaviour Therapy and Experimental Psychiatry*, vol. 7 (1976), pp. 285–8.

18. Meichenbaum, D.H. *Cognitive Behaviour Modification* (New York, Plenum Press, 1975).

19. Meichenbaum, D.H. and Goodman, J. 'Training impulsive children to talk to themselves', *Journal of Abnormal Psychology*, vol. 77 (1971), pp. 115–26.

20. Novaco, R.W. *Anger Control: The Development and Evaluation of an Experimental Treatment* (Lexington, Mass., Heath, 1975).

21. Horan, J.T., Hackett, G., Nichanan, J.D., Stone, C.I. and Stone, D.D. 'Coping with pain: a component analysis of stress inoculation', *Cognitive Therapy and Research*, vol. 1, no. 3 (1977), pp. 211–21.

22. Russell, R.K. and Sipich, J.F. 'Cue-controlled relaxation in the treatment of test anxiety', *Journal of Behaviour Therapy and Experimental Psychiatry*, vol. 4 (1973), pp. 47–9.

23. Ellis, A. and Harper, R.A. *A Guide to Rational Living* (N. Hollywood, California, Wilshire, 1961).

24. Ellis, A. (ed.) *Growth through Reason* (Palo Alto, California, Science and Behavior Books, 1971).

25. Beck, A.T. *Cognitive Therapy and the Emotional Disorders* (New York, International Universities Press, 1976).

26. For detailed description of CT see: Beck, A.T., Rush, A.J., Shaw, B.F. and Emery, G. *Cognitive Therapy of Depression* (New York, Wiley, 1980).

27. Ablett, I. 'Phobias in a case of manic-depressive psychosis', *CCNS Course Reports* (unpublished report, Royal Dundee Liff Hospital, 1981).

9 BEHAVIOURAL GROUP THERAPY

> Only a beast or a god is fit to live alone.
> — Aristotle

Group or Individual Treatment

In the last two chapters a range of behaviour-change techniques was discussed. Some have had wide-ranging success, while others show more modest results with a more limited range of problems. The need to select treatment methods with a good 'track record' has been stressed repeatedly. We have also argued that the nurse may, on many occasions, need to design a treatment package which is geared to the special needs of her patient. In this chapter we shall pursue treatment one stage further, by considering the role of established treatment packages. These programmes, which include a number of the individual techniques which have been discussed, are designed to tackle broad problem areas and may often be applied in either individual or group treatment settings. In concluding this section on behavour-change methods, we shall consider the problem 'areas' highlighted by the three patients whom we met earlier in the book. We shall also discuss the kind of treatment packages which might prove beneficial for these patients and their specific problems of living.

Social Behaviour

Most people would argue that individual treatment is preferable to treatment in groups, especially where a specialised service is provided to meet the special needs of the patient. The close relationship with the nurse, which the patient enjoys in individualised care, may also enhance the effect of the specific treatment methods used. In many instances, however, group treatment may be necessary purely for economic reasons. In such a situation treatment will, of necessity, be more impersonal and less oriented towards the specific needs of the individual. In other cases, treatment in a group setting may be necessary to resolve some aspect of the problem. This is often the case with problems involving social behaviour.

Primary and Secondary Groups. Many of the problems illustrated in our short case histories in Chapter 3 involve social behaviour. Mrs Smith's anxiety is centred upon specific social situations and her depression is largely a function of difficult interactions with other people, especially her mother and husband. Sally is seen as socially disruptive or unsociable. Brian's lack of self-care and social skills would cause him few difficulties in a more primitive, less socialised, culture. However, apart from the hermit or the lighthouse keeper, most people are obliged to spend a large proportion of their lives in one social grouping or another. This is very true of our three 'patient' stereotypes. We label them as problematic or deviant, if they break certain social conventions, or the patient may feel that he has a problem if he cannot live up to the rules which he has set himself, regarding his ability to deal with other people. Whether we assess ourselves or are assessed by others, social competence is seen as an important measure of our overall 'personal effectiveness'.

Sociologists distinguish between the different social groups to which we may belong. *Primary groups* are made up of our friends, family and daily associates or acquaintances. *Secondary groups* are made up of people we interact with — like the bus driver or shopkeeper, whom we have never met before and may never meet again. In primary groups, our interactions are close and intimate. In secondary groups, relationships are more formal and are characterised by greater social distance. Primary groups serve an important function. Here we find companionship, mutual support, the chance to discuss our problems and to learn from others. Loyalties are strongest in the primary group, in which we also find most of our social satisfactions. The person with limited primary-group contact may lack a sense of 'belonging'; and may be ill-equipped to deal with the stress of everyday life. Durkhaim, the French sociologist, showed that suicide was highest amongst those whose primary-group ties were weakest.

The need to build, or strengthen, social behaviour is a high priority for all the patients we have discussed so far. The problems experienced by someone like Mrs Smith suggest that she is unable to gain the social support which she needs. On the other hand, the antisocial behaviour of patients like Brian and Sally may prejudice future, or sever existing, links with family or friends. The treatment programme, for all three patients, would emphasise the need to increase or establish appropriate social, or pro-social, skills.

The Benefits of Group Treatment.   Traditionally, the decision to treat patients in groups has been an expedient one: inadequate resources have often been the stimulus for 'block treatment'. Ideally, the decision to run a group programme should be based upon the needs of the patient, rather than upon economics. Although some problems can be dealt with *only* in a group setting, others may benefit when group exposure is arranged as an adjunct to individual programming. Even where the treatment programme is wholly patient-centred, the ultimate goal of therapy may be 'social effectiveness', in one form or another.

The benefits of group treatment can be seen from the patient's or the nurse's viewpoint. The group will offer the patient:

(1) The moral support of patients experiencing similar problems.
(2) An opportunity to discuss and practise solutions to his problems, through role-play.
(3) A chance to learn from others through modelling.
(4) An opportunity to strengthen existing interpersonal skills, through meeting and interacting with others on a regular basis.
(5) A guaranteed level of nurse–patient interaction. This may be an important consideration for the patient in hospital.
(6) A consistent therapeutic relationship with a range of nurses. Where nurses rotate around various groups, the patient may gain the help of different nurses, all of whom will use the same therapeutic approach.

The group will offer the nurse:

(1) A practical way of providing effective care to a range of patients, especially where the programme is linked to existing routines.
(2) A range of patient contacts within one programme: this may increase 'job satisfaction'.
(3) A reduction in stress. For many nurses, one-to-one relationships can be very demanding.
(4) An opportunity to manipulate peer-group pressure, particularly when working with difficult patients. This strategy may also help reduce stress by locating 'authority' within the group.
(5) An ideal situation to train new staff. Nurses may participate in the group – and study its processes – as a member, before taking the responsibility of running the session.

Composition of the Group. Groups should be composed of patients with similar problems, which handicap each member more or less to the same extent. Unless they are a primary group already, the nurse should group patients according to age and social and cultural background, except where this would be inappropriate. This may help promote 'togetherness' or group cohesion. Patients who are *less* disabled than the rest of the group may be included and may prove useful models for their peers. However, patients who are much *more* disabled than the majority may feel that they cannot compete and may be sorely disadvantaged.

Mixed-sex groups are recommended, except where this would be inappropriate, e.g. in dressing or toiletting programmes. Although the size of the group depends upon the number of nurses participating, in general groups of ten or more are not recommended. Where close attention needs to be paid to individuals during the session — in the form of observation or instruction — the group may be much smaller. In general, the size of the group is determined by the time available and how this needs to be allocated, e.g. the time required for role-play or setting homework assignments.

Cost-effectiveness. Even where problems are not strictly social or inter-personal, patients can benefit from group treatment. Group desensitisa-tion, where patients with similar fears are treated with a common hierarchy, is one area which has been studied closely. In other studies, patients have constructed their own hierarchies, writing this on a card for reference and responding to the group leader's instruction to 'imagine the scene described on card one'. Group desensitisation has been shown to be more effective than traditional group treatment, where height phobics and claustrophobics were involved.[1] Other researchers have shown that spider phobics, public-speaking phobics, snake phobics, and those with anxiety in 'test' situations[2] also benefit from treatment in behavioural groups. In a wider context, Kazdin[3] has discussed the contribution of treatment of a wide range of patients in token economy groups. These studies illustrate the cost-effectiveness of group treatment, one therapist being able to deliver treatment to a number of patients all at the same time.

The Case for Individual Treatment. Problems which are social in charac-ter, but which do not involve social interaction, such as eating, dressing and grooming, may be difficult to manage within a group context. Although these behaviours may be shown in the company of others (like eating) or may be part of the patient's social image (like grooming) they are performed independently. Although these *pro-social* skills can be dealt with in a group setting, the individual attention which the patient may require may nullify the value of the group exercise.

Even where problems are wholly social in nature, the patient may reject the offer of group treatment. He may be unwilling to discuss his problem in front of others, even when they share the same difficulties. The patient may wish to maintain the security of an individual programme, where his privacy is assured. In the case of certain problems, such as severe depression, it may not be possible to translate treatment techniques for use in group settings. In the situations mentioned above the nurse must arrange individual therapy: to suit the nature of the problem, to fulfil the patient's wishes or to make use of the most appropriate change-techniques.

Behavioural Group Therapy

From consideration of the issues raised so far, a *range* of group treatments appears possible. In some cases the nature of the problem may demand treatment in a social context. Various group processes, such as modelling effects, mutual support and group identity, may make a significant contribution to the success of the therapy. For such problems 'treatment-*through*-groups' is indicated.

Where patients share common problems, which are not interpersonal in character, one 'therapist' may treat a number of patients using a common programme or one with slight modifications to suit the individuals in the group. Where cost-effectiveness is an important consideration, 'treatment-*in*-groups' may be indicated.

Where the patient has major deficits in pro-social behaviour, treatment in a group setting may be contra-indicated. Here the patient needs individual attention to help eliminate antisocial behaviour or acquire basic skills. However, in the intermediate and later stages of the programme social exposure will be arranged to test out the generalisability of the patient's new skills. In this situation 'treatment-*for*-groups' is indicated.

We shall now illustrate each of these distinct behavioural group therapies, using our case stereotypes as examples.

Treatment through Groups: Advanced Social Skills

Social Anxiety

Mrs Smith listed a number of problems of living which, by her account, revolve around anxiety and depression. Here we shall consider a treatment approach which focuses upon her 'unassertiveness'. We shall take the view that this may be a central problem for this patient. Although separate treatment programmes could be arranged for anxiety, depression and assertiveness, here we shall try to kill three birds with one stone.

Assertion Deficit. On interview, Mrs Smith revealed two facets of her assertion deficit: she cannot argue effectively with her mother and has great difficulty in expressing her feelings. Since her marriage foundered recently, a similar problem may have existed in her relationship with her husband. Assertive behaviour is an honest and straightforward expression of thoughts and feelings. When a person is assertive, he behaves in a socially appropriate manner, taking the feelings of others into account. This means that assertion and *aggression* are poles apart. The aggressive person expresses his feelings in an unacceptable manner, without taking the other person into consideration. Assertion can be conceptualised as the mid-point between passivity and aggression. Patients who are passive and submissive, however, often complain of 'explosive rages' when they are 'pushed too far'. In Mrs Smith's case, when she can tolerate her mother's overbearing attitude no further, she communicates this only obliquely by taking a drug overdose.

Anxiety and Assertion. Mrs Smith stressed that her anxiety was confined largely to social and interpersonal situations. Inability to express negative feelings (such as anger, jealousy or resentment) or positive feelings (such as love or praise) can often lead to anxiety. Mrs Smith becomes particularly anxious when confronted by a shopkeeper, her boss or her mother, who criticises, abuses or manipulates her. If she could defend herself, by saying 'No', or by asking that *her* rights and views be respected, she would be under little or no threat. As she cannot do this she becomes 'putty in other people's hands'. She has learned to cope with such situations by escaping from them or by avoiding them altogether. A man who gets flustered when asking a woman for a date, or who gets tongue-tied when asking his boss for a raise, or who blushes and stutters when retorting to the jibes of a teenage gang, is experiencing a similar kind of problem. He may suffer anticipatory anxiety, each time such a situation looms on the horizon. By escaping or avoiding these situations, he maintains the power of such events to evoke anxiety. The frustration which results can lead to the kind of depression described by Mrs Smith, when the patient reflects on 'how spineless, weak-willed or pathetic I am'.

Selection of Patients. In Mrs Smith's case we may assume that her social phobia, depression and lack of assertion are related. We are not saying that all patients with social anxiety and depression have assertion problems. In the same way we should not assume that the unassertive patient is an obvious 'personality type'. Unassertive patients are often stereotyped as meek, shy-looking individuals who cannot say boo to a goose. Some patients may in fact be assertive in one situation (e.g. at work) but quite ineffectual in another (e.g. at home). Similarly many patients appear confident on interview, smiling and talking with no obvious show of anxiety. This may, however, be only a superficial image which cracks under the stress of particular interpersonal relationships. Four classes of patient may benefit from assertion training:

(1) The patient who is unable to express positive feelings in a socially acceptable manner.
(2) The patient who is showing signs that he is blocking the expression of some intense emotion, such as anger or jealousy.
(3) The patient who suffers from interpersonal anxiety.
(4) The patient who habitually avoids important social events.

In each of these cases, unassertiveness should be interpreted as a behavioural deficit and *not* as a personality trait.

In addition to these categories are patients who complain that they are socially 'incompetent', but on observation appear to be as competent as the next person. For such patients, cognitive restructuring, to modify their self-perception, may be indicated. A second contradiction is the patient who believes that he functions well in company, but is upset to find that he is constantly rebuffed or criticised. This patient may need specific help to recognise the aspects of his behaviour which upset other people and to learn some alternatives.

The History of Assertion Training

Salter first described 'assertion training' in the late 1940s when he discussed the use of excitatory exercises to overcome a number of psychological problems.[4] These involved:

(1) The use of feeling talk: patients practised expressing both positive and negative feelings.
(2) The use of facial talk: patients practised using facial expression to accompany particular emotional expressions.
(3) The expression of contradictory opinions.
(4) Practising agreeing with a compliment.
(5) Practising improvising within conversations.

The first major application of assertion training was by Wolpe.[5] Instead of doling out assertion training to all patients, as Salter had done, Wolpe tried to identify patients who appeared to need this approach. He noted that some patients could be assertive with, for example, their family but not with their employers. He concluded that assertion was a behavioural asset and not a personality trait. Wolpe also paid close attention to the consequences of assertive behaviour in his treatment programmes. He appreciated that he could easily court disaster by practising his new-found skills in a hostile environment. He stressed, therefore, the need to encourage the patient towards his final assertive goal through gradual stages, using the principles of systematic desensitisation. Another significant contribution to assertive training was made by Albert Ellis, who described the identification of self-defeating thoughts which are associated with unassertive behaviour. Therapists have built more 'cognitive' considerations into the treatment programme in recent years, allowing the patient to tackle the irrational thoughts and beliefs which feed his assertion deficit.

Presenting the Programme

The nurse's first task is to explain her reasons for selecting this approach and to try to gain the patient's approval. If Mrs Smith is dubious about the group aspect of treatment, a few individual sessions might be offered, after which one, two and then three or more patients would be included. This simple strategy would desensitise her to the fear of 'the group'. The first question the patient may ask, if only of herself, is 'What good is all this going to do me?' Although some authors suggest that the patient should be encouraged to think that she has a *right* to be assertive, from the very outset, this may cause complications. If Mrs Smith assumes that this means that she should *always* be assertive, she may criticise and punish herself, whenever she fails to meet this standard. As an alternative, the nurse might suggest that the patient will gain benefits by being assertive. She may point out that although it is not 'wrong' to be unassertive, such behaviour is, by its very nature, self-defeating. The nurse should not force her view on to the patient, but should highlight examples where the patient's behaviour has resulted in personal losses or upset. She may suggest, further, that the patient has nothing to lose by trying assertion training. A brief summary of the case of a patient, who benefited from this approach, may be one of the best ways of introducing the therapy to the patient. This illustration may encourage the patient to follow the example of a 'fellow sufferer'. The nurse could also give a summary of the aims of assertion training: being able to say 'No' when someone makes an unreasonable request; expressing feelings, both positive and negative; making reasonable requests of other people; and initiating and carry-ing on conversations. In order to express the overall aim of treatment, the nurse might discuss therapy in terms of a 'social skills training' exercise.[6]

The Training Session

The group should comprise of five to eight patients and two nurses, one to act as group leader and the other as co-therapist. The group should meet for one to one-and-a-half hours in a comfortable setting, at least once a week. Each session will be devoted to analysing individual problems, identifying possible solutions and practising these through role-play. At the end of each session each member is given a homework assignment which he will 'report back' upon at the next session.

Introduction.   The first session concentrates upon introducing the patients to each other and to the assertion training model. Each patient is asked to say something to a neighbour. This behaviour, like the assertive response which follows later, is modelled by the group leader, who opens the session:

> *Leader:* Okay, just to get the group warmed up I'd like us all to introduce ourselves. Tell everyone what you would like to be called in the group, and tell us a little bit about yourself. Okay? Well . . . I'm Angela. I'm . . . about thirty (laughs) and I'm married with a little boy. I'm going to take the session for the next few weeks. (nods to patient on immediate right)
> *Patient:* Err . . . my name is Dave. I come from Fenwood. I'm twenty-seven. I've got these problems with people see . . . I just can't seem to . . .
> *Leader:* That's fine Dave. You spoke up very well. We'll come back to the details of your problem, a little later on. Good. Okay? (nods to patient on immediate left)

In this introduction 'game' the nurse tries to set the mood for the rest of the group. She gives each patient a chance to say a few words, encouraging each one no matter how tongue-tied he may become. She will also discourage patients like Dave from beginning a 'confession', since this is not on the agenda and will add to the other patients' anxiety. When modelling, the nurses present a warm and friendly image.

They avoid appearing knowledgeable or too articulate as this may inhibit patients who are already feeling anxious. A second 'round' can be added where the patients are invited to ask each other a simple question. 'How are you today? Have you been here before? How far is it from Fenwood on the bus? Once again the nurses shape up the patient's interpersonal style, praising the patient's eye-contact, tone of voice, etc., even where this is poor. She will then suggest that he tries to improve this good feature, next time around.

Pleasantries and Positive Self-talk.   In the next round the patients are asked to pay a compliment to someone in the room. Again, this is modelled by the leader: the co-therapist adds further modelling at the mid-point of the round, to prevent the compliments becoming too stereotyped. The nurses continue to shape more confident speech, prompting each patient to attend to the important non-verbal signs of eye-contact and posture. The group are asked next to make positive self-statements aloud: owning up to a particular skill or identifying their favourite hobby, etc.

Conversation.   In the final phase of this first session the group practise making *small talk* – discussing the weather, the bus trip to the clinic, or an item from the newspaper – and finally, *breaking into* conversation – where two patients are chatting and a third must 'join in' at an appropriate pause. These last two exercises are the patients' first experience of the assertion-training format, where they will act out a situation with one or two other patients, as the rest of the group observe. Since this is the first session, the nurses must lavish the patients with praise, whether justified or not, to ease their anxiety and to ensure that they return the following week. In winding up the session the nurses will invite another round of evaluative comments:

> *Leader:* Okay, that's the first session nearly over. How did you think it went, Wendy?
> *Wendy:* Oh, well . . . I was pretty nervous at first . . . I still am . . . but I think it was worthwhile . . . I mean . . . I . . .
> *Leader:* Good, Wendy, I'm glad that you feel that you got something from this first session. I felt that you were making a real effort. That's great. I'll look forward to seeing how you get on next week. What about you, Walter. Any thoughts about tonight's session?

Role Play and Role Reversal

At the next session the leader asks each patient to describe his problem, encouraging him to define this in terms of his behaviour in specific situations (see Figure 9.1). The assertion training session then begins:

(1) The patient is asked to act out the situation with a partner from the group. Mrs Smith might ask someone to play her mother, having described how she usually acts in the 'problem situation'.

(2) The nurse then gives the patient some feedback on her performance in the role play. 'That was good . . . I liked the way you tried to look at her . . . you didn't turn away completely. How about if you tried it again. This time you might . . .' The feedback must be positive and constructive, never punitive. Most of all the nurse must appear friendly and understanding.

(3) The nurse models briefly (1–2 minutes) some of the key points of a more assertive response, stressing both verbal and non-verbal communication. She strives not to appear too competent.

(4) The patient repeats the role play (approximately two minutes).

(5) The nurse reinforces strongly any slight improvement: asking the patient to repeat sections of the role play briefly to strengthen facets of the assertive response. If she finds imitation of the modelled response difficult, role reversal may be employed. Mrs Smith would be asked to take her mother's part, while another patient played her part in the interaction.

Leader: Nora (Mrs Smith) has told us that she is having problems with her mother. Let's see how she usually handles her mother and her bossy nature. Nora . . . who would you like to work with you on this?

Nora: I'm not sure. What about Sally? (the co-therapist) Would that be okay?

Leader: Fine. Sally, you be mother. You're giving Nora some advice about 'straightening herself out'. Nora, show us how you'd handle it. (Role play follows: two to three minutes)

Leader: Fine, let's just cut it there. How did you feel, Nora?

Nora: Oh that was just me. I seem to go along with her. Anything to shut her up. Even though we were just acting I still feel pretty tense.

Leader: That's okay, Nora. (to group) Anyone like to comment? (pause)

Sally: Well, I thought it wasn't too bad. I see what Nora means

Figure 9.1: Nurses Prompt and Reinforce during Role Play

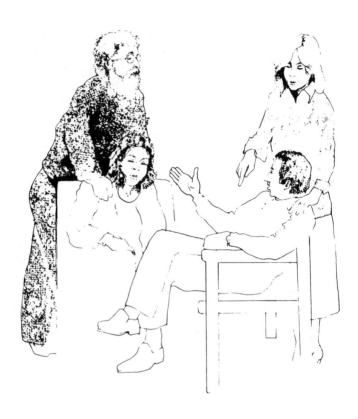

about her getting tense. I got the impression at first that she was trying to resist me a bit. Then, as soon as I cut in again she just gave in and started agreeing with me.

Nora: You're right of course. I just don't know what to say to her.

Leader: Look Nora, it's obvious that you've a good idea of what you *ought* to be doing. How about if you tightened up on that 'resistance' a bit for starters? Try looking at her — full in the face —

and saying, 'I'm sorry Mum, I'm a bit busy now' or perhaps 'I understand what you're trying to say, but I just don't see things that way'. Maybe Sally could take your part this time and you could play your mother, just to see what we mean?

Verbal and Non-verbal Behaviour.   After this role reversal Mrs Smith would take her own part again, modelling herself on Sally's example. The leader encourages the group to pick out the strengths and weaknesses of her performance, perhaps using a visual aid, such as a blackboard, to emphasise the important features of assertive behaviour. Although most unassertive people complain of their lack of fluency or speech content, we communicate as much with our bodies, as we do with our voices. Anxiety, shyness, anger, etc., are often shown by how we act, rather than by what we say. This should be pointed out to the group, emphasising that the patient can become more effective by making simple changes in specific non-verbal behaviours.

Eye-contact: the patient must learn to give appropriate eye-contact (or gaze). In normal interaction this means looking at the other person approximately 75 per cent of the time. Looking downwards, or away from the person, often means 'I am shy or frightened'. Staring, or gazing more than 75 per cent of the time means 'I am confronting you or I am angry'.

Facial expression: the patient should be shown how to use his face to display, or illustrate, his irritation, or happiness, etc.

Posture and gestures: the patient should be shown how different ways of 'posing' the body also display different moods. Standing upright with his head held high means 'I am confident'. A sprawling posture when seated means 'I am comfortable and relaxed'. He is also shown how to use appropriate gestures to help 'describe' or 'emphasise' what he is saying.

Orientation: the patient's physical relationship to the other person also says much about how he is feeling. Standing close with his body turned 'full face' to the other person may mean 'I am confronting you with this issue, I am not going to give in'. Standing sideways to the other person with his head slightly averted may mean 'I appreciate that I was wrong but . . .'

Speech content also varies according to the demands of the situation. Once again, however, some general principles about the use of the voice can be given.

Latency: the time which the patient takes to answer the other person is of crucial importance. If he hurries his replies he may appear anxious. If he is too slow, he may appear uninterested. Examples of the situations in which instant replies or slightly delayed reactions will be to his advantage, should be illustrated.

Duration: where the patient is anxious his speeches may be very short or may tend to trail off. Gradual lengthening of speeches, using a shaping procedure, should be demonstrated. At the same time the benefits of short, abrupt statements in certain situations should be modelled.

Tone: one danger of all social skills training approaches is that the patient may model himself too closely on the trainer and may end up speaking like a robot. The nurse should emphasise the need to sound happy, or angry, etc. She should also demonstrate simple relaxation procedures to overcome sounding 'high-pitched' when anxious and how to avoid muttering and mumbling when passive.

Assertion as 'Normal' Behaviour.   In all sessions the nurse must be aware of the social and cultural background of the patient. In order for assertive behaviour to be *appropriate* it must be adapted to suit specific social settings. Two other assertion, and general social skills, training approaches are worthy of mention in this respect. Goldstein[7] has produced a package called Structured Learning Therapy which is geared specifically towards the needs of chronic psychiatric patients and the mentally handicapped. A similar approach developed by Liberman[8] is called Personal Effectiveness. This approach has been used with a wide variety of patients who present with a range of social and interpersonal problems. With both approaches the need to help the patient learn appropriate social behaviour is heavily emphasised.

The Use of Other Techniques.   The assertion training group can also incorporate other techniques. Some practitioners favour beginning the session with group relaxation to overcome the anxiety which patients may experience on entering the group. Others use modifications of the stress management or cognitive methods discussed in Chapter 8. These more sophisticated techniques would be introduced at later stages of the programme, when the patient has become more active in solving his own problems.

Summary

Mrs Smith's problems of living involve her reactions to everyday events, like her mother's 'domineering' behaviour, which need not produce emotional difficulties. The assertion training group aims to help her cope more effectively with these everyday stresses. The group offers her an opportunity to practise solutions to her problems, in an atmosphere of mutual support. The problems may be arranged in a hierarchy to maximise the chances of success, beginning with the less severe and progressing over several weeks or months to tackle her most difficult situations. The nurse acts as a model for the patient in the early stages of role play, passing this task on to the patient's peers in gradual stages. More assertive responses are 'shaped up' by providing positive feedback and helpful suggestions, rather than criticism. Homework assignments are planned carefully in advance of each session and are aimed at giving the patient a chance to practise her assertive behaviour in a real-life situation. These assignments are graded carefully to provide the patient with the greatest chance of success in the early stages and to ensure that she does not meet potentially aversive 'conflicts' until she is better equipped to deal with them.

Treatment-in-Groups: Basic Social Skills

Antisocial Behaviour

Sally's problems involve social behaviour of a wholly different order. She is unco-operative and can be aggressive, both physically and verbally, with staff and patients alike. She spends much of her waking day begging for cigarettes and is loathe to participate in the self-care and social routines of the ward. Had she not been admitted to the ward only recently, we might have assumed that she had never been 'socialised'. Her diagnosis of Korsakoff's psychosis indicates the presence of brain damage. Staff who complain that they cannot reason with her as 'it doesn't sink in' may well be struggling with massive memory defect. Sally's problems could be categorised as follows:

(1) Self-care deficits: she does not eat an adequate diet and is poorly motivated to bathe or attend to her appearance.
(2) Aggressive outbursts: she loses her temper when thwarted and may use violence to solve interpersonal conflict.
(3) 'Antisocial' behaviour: she often walks around partially undressed and swears profusely. She is most infamous, however, for begging cigarettes from all-and-sundry.
(4) Apathy: much of her free time is spent dozing in an armchair. She resists passively attempts to engage her in conversation or games, etc.

As with Mrs Smith, these problems could be dealt with separately. However, individual programming on such a scale on a long-term ward would be very costly in terms of staff time. A group programme, within which Sally's problems could be tackled specifically, would be the most practical solution. Since Sally has developed her own style of coping with the ups and downs of ward life, she is unlikely to wish to change her lifestyle radically. The treatment programme will, therefore, need to be built around the idea of motivating Sally, over a long period, to behave in a more socially acceptable manner.

The Token Economy

Any treatment programme which can cover all four problem areas will be complex. Since it will be concerned mainly with promoting one class of behaviour and reducing another, it will emphasise the use of contingency management techniques. The *token economy* was first described in depth by Ayllon and Azrin[9] as a motivational system for therapy and rehabilitation. The system showed that even chronically institutionalised patients could be helped to lead more productive lives, through a treatment programme which was not over-costly in staff time or expertise. Although the system is concerned mainly with strengthening or weakening *existing* behaviour, skills training can be included. Since Sally's behaviour repertoire is not wholly maladaptive, the programme would encourage her to show more of her (currently limited) appropriate behaviour and less of her socially embarrassing behaviour. Where she appears to be lacking totally in skills — such as anger control — specific training might be needed to establish such behaviour from scratch.

Token Programmes. In the token *economy* a wide range of behaviours are treated in a group setting. This often takes place as part of an existing routine: ward activities, a school day or the domestic routine of a hostel. In the token *system* one person, or a very small group, is treated for only one or two problems. In this situation tokens are used only as expedient reinforcers in a programme which emphasises other treatment or training methods. A token economy would be indicated for Sally since she has many problems, some of which might benefit from exposure within a large group setting.

Advantages and Disadvantages. The token economy offers a chance to tackle a range of problems within the context of the patient's everyday routine. Other advantages are:

(1) A large number of patients may be included. The programme may be a 'blanket' one, where all patients have the same targets and receive the same token contingencies. In a 'streamed' programme a number of sub-groups contain patients at different levels of ability on the same targets. The programme may also be individualised, so that each patient is on his own treatment schedule, which operates within a group context.

(2) The programme can include as many areas of behaviour as the staff can handle. In Sally's case the programme would have four main areas: improving self-care, increasing social and pro-social skills, increasing recreational activity and planning and carrying out her own daily routine.

(3) Tokens do not interfere with the performance of a chain of behaviours. If Sally was given a cigarette as a reinforcer for washing herself, smoking this 'reinforcer' would interfere with the chain of grooming behaviours. Within the token economy Sally can collect tokens at various points in the grooming chain and exchange them later for back-up reinforcers (e.g. a cigarette with a cup of tea at mid-morning).

(4) The same token can be used to reinforce a range of patients with widely different reinforcement preferences.

(5) There is no limit to the number of token reinforcers which the patient can accumulate. Since the patient can spend some tokens and bank others, for future reinforcement, the risk of satiation is reduced.

(6) The token economy can manipulate back-up reinforcers which would not be available under a standard contingency management programme. The token 'bridges the gap' between the behaviour and access to the back-up reinforcer. 'Shaving in the morning' can, as a result, be reinforced by 'going to the cinema at night'.

(7) The economy can be inflated or deflated according to the capabilities of the patient. Early in the programme one token may buy one cigarette. Later, two, three or even ten tokens may be required for the same cigarette, as the patient finds it easier to earn tokens. This principle of pricing applies in everyday life, as every shopper knows.

(8) One token can buy a small portion of a reinforcer. A visit to the Old Tyme Music Hall might cost forty tokens. Combing her hair might, therefore, be reinforced by a very small part of this desired back-up reinforcer.

(9) The possession of tokens can cue other staff to give extra social approval.

(10) Through their association with the delivery of tokens, staff may

become more socially reinforcing. This is important when tokens are phased out and the patient's gains are maintained by social contingencies alone.

The token economy also has some disadvantages:

(1) The reinforcement system is not the same as that which prevails in the natural community. Although patients who are institutionalised permanently are not adversely affected by this, rehabilitation patients must be weaned off the system before discharge.

(2) Institutions often find it difficult to maintain the store of back-up reinforcers. This is especially so if staff do not wish to use everyday reinforcers, such as watching TV, sweets, etc. – which they consider to be the patient's rights.

(3) Some patients need to be taught, or re-taught, the value of a currency system. This is often the case with mentally handicapped people or chronic psychiatric patients who have had limited contact with everyday currency systems.

(4) Since patients are rarely at the same level of ability it may be necessary to individualise the programme. Where each patient has a different set of 'rules' for targets and reinforcement, management of the programme becomes much more complex.

The Basis of the Economy.   The token economy has three characteristics which must be defined before the programme can begin:

(1) *The Target Behaviours.*   Some behaviours will be targets for increase, others for decrease. Tokens may be given (positive reinforcement) for eating breakfast or talking appropriately, and taken away (response cost) for asking for cigarettes, shouting and swearing.

(2) *The Token Currency.*   A variety of tokens may be used. Plastic counters, points on a tally sheet, gummed stars on a wallboard, or holes punched in a card carried by the patient, are all possibilities. The only condition is that the patient understands the role of the token.

(3) *The Exchange Rate.*   A reinforcement 'menu' comprising of all the back-up items and activity reinforcers, should be prepared. This should detail how many tokens may be exchanged for these reinforcers.

Organisation of the Programme

The token economy is a complex social system. Patients like Sally are living in a bustling social setting, where 'rules' are written, broken, rewritten and interpreted loosely, from one day to the next. If the token economy is to have the slightest chance of success the following rules must be enforced.

Control over Reinforcers.   The items and activities included on the 'menu' must be available *only* in exchange for tokens. This means that staff, relatives and other patients must be discouraged from providing free or non-contingent reinforcement. This control is often difficult to establish since staff and relatives often believe that these reinforcers are the patient's by right. This is an ethical judgement which must be debated during the initial planning stage of the programme. The clear aim of the programme is to 'motivate' Sally and other patients towards a more independent and socially appropriate lifestyle. If manipulation of such everyday reinforcers can help achieve this, then controlled access may be justified.

Staff Co-ordination.   Where a treatment programme operates across the patients' waking day, a number of different staff will be involved. To ensure that each nurse handles each patient in much the same way, strict guidelines regarding nurse–patient interaction may need to be enforced. In particular, nurses must be advised against making even minor changes in the programme. The nursing policy must dictate procedures for observing patients, recording their behaviour, giving and withdrawing tokens, the criteria for deciding upon 'appropriate' and 'inappropriate' behaviour, when tokens may be exchanged and the current exchange rates. These guidelines must be strictly adhered to if all patients are to have the maximum opportunity to learn the new 'rules' which govern behaviour on the ward.

Defining Target Behaviours.   In many token economies the objective may be to stop the patient performing some unacceptable behaviour. In Sally's case we might want her to stop being aggressive, pestering others for cigarettes, avoiding routines, etc. It is often difficult to achieve such *negative* goals. It is easier to suggest positive targets, such as 'arguing a point without shouting and swearing', 'budgetting your cigarette allocation', 'completing your daily routines'. Although it is still important to reduce her antisocial behaviour, Sally is learning *what to do*, rather than simply what not to do.

Identifying Appropriate Reinforcers.   In Chapter 4 we discussed how we could draw up the patient's reinforcement menu. In Sally's case there may be a scarcity of positive reinforcers. Staff might only be able to identify basic reinforcers, such as sitting in a favourite armchair, smoking or going early to bed. Institutionalised patients often value only a small range of reinforcers, often avoiding activities which we view as reinforcing. Ayllon and Azrin described how very regressed patients could be introduced to a wider range of reinforcers through a *sampling* procedure. Initially none of the patients was willing to pay tokens to 'go for a walk outside', 'sit in the music room' or 'watch a film show'. Staff then encouraged the patients to sample the activity by assembling them outside, leaving the music room door ajar, or by letting them watch five minutes of the film, before asking if the patient wished to pay tokens for the rest of the reinforcer. Many of the patients bought the rest of the reinforcer after sampling it; this continued long after the sampling procedure had stopped. In the case of patients like Sally, such a sampling procedure might be very worthwhile, as a means of widening her range of reinforcers.

Token Awards and Exchanges.   The nursing policy must define clearly how many tokens are given or taken away for each behaviour. Those behaviours which the patient finds easy, or which she already performs to a limited extent, will be awarded fewer tokens than those which she does not do at all. Sally might receive twenty tokens each time she answers a question in a group discussion, but only two or three for spending ten minutes washing dishes. The number of tokens is determined by the likelihood that the patient will perform the behaviour. Exchange rates are determined by demand. Those items or activities which the patient asks for most often will require a larger number of tokens than those which he is less likely to ask for. Supply, as well as demand, will influence the token 'charges'. A trip to town may not be valued all that highly, but may be difficult to organise. This would make it an expensive reinforcer. In some cases the cost of certain reinforcers may be reduced to increase the patient's engagement in the activity: e.g. the cost of 'talking to staff' or 'a tin of talcum powder' may be kept very low, to increase Sally's social interaction and personal hygiene behaviours.

Fading of Tokens.   The token economy is an artificial way of motivating the patient. Although it is similar to a bonus system in industry, it is not the way people usually acquire social or pro-social skills. More important, it differs markedly from the system which controls social behaviour in the community. It is important, therefore, that patients are weaned off the programme as preparation for discharge into the community. This may be done by *delaying* the delivery of token: instead of giving tokens at each stage of, for example, the grooming process, these may be given as soon as grooming is completed. Reinforcement may be delayed further until a 'grooming-check' at mid-morning and mid-afternoon, and then to a check at random times during the day, and finally at random points during the week. The patient continues performing the behaviour in anticipation of reinforcement which appears on a variable schedule. Alternatively, the number of tokens given for each target behaviour can be reduced gradually. Sally might gain ten tokens for brushing her hair in the first phase of the programme. This will be reduced gradually over a period of weeks or even months, as she becomes more proficient. At the same time the 'buying power' of tokens can be increased, as the number of available tokens decreases.

Social Reinforcement. It is of vital importance that social approval is given each time tokens are delivered. Although Sally may not value this initially, these 'approving' comments may become conditioned reinforcers through their association with tokens. When the tokens are being phased out the social approval is still given. For instance, when Sally speaks at a group meeting, although no tokens are given the nurse might say, 'Yes, that's very true Sally. Nice to hear you speaking up. What did the rest of you think of that point which Sally just made?' At a grooming check the nurse might say, 'I really like the way you've done your hair Sally. It looks really smashing. Maybe you can show me how you did it, later on perhaps?' Although there has been little research on the fading of tokens, studies have shown that the performance of pro-social skills does not drop off, when tokens are faded gradually.[10]

Presenting the Programme to the Patient

The token economy is largely a staff-controlled affair. The patient is engineered towards certain targets. If access to highly valued reinforcers is not controlled, Sally will be unlikely to change her behaviour. However, this does not mean that staff should not try to involve the patient in the programme. Indeed, it is important that all aspects of the proposed programme are discussed with her, at least as a warning of the impending change in ward policy. Where possible, the nurse should try to enlist some small degree of support from the patient.

Individual Differences. Although it is not clear from our summary how communicative Sally is likely to be, the nurse should take some time to explain the programme to her, giving her some examples of how it will operate in practice and what benefits she might gain from the programme. Since Sally suffers from some degree of memory impairment, the programme would emphasise the use of repeated instructions, visual aids in parts of the ward and repeated feedback to the patient as soon as she has performed 'appropriate' or 'inappropriate' behaviour. In a study with a patient with Korsakoff's psychosis McFadden[11] used notices written in simple language and very large letters, which were fixed to the wall above the patient's bed, in the toilet area, kitchen, etc. These acted as reminders at various times in the day. The patient was oriented to each notice, and the programme did not begin until she could explain what it said and how it related to her own behaviour. This patient also showed the kind of cigarette-begging which Sally displays. A large record form was fixed to the wall in the nursing station. Each time the patient asked for a cigarette, the nurse recorded this on a tally counter and recorded the total each hour. At various points in the day the patient was taken to the nursing station and shown her chart. If her 'requests' had not exceeded a set limit, she was given a number of tokens. If she exceeded the limit, the tokens were deposited in a response-cost box. The 'request limit' was set, initially, at a level at which she could be successful; this was decreased gradually so that her begging behaviour would be reduced accordingly.

In a study by Portues[12] the patient carried her own record sheet at each stage in the programme. Each time the programme was adjusted to increase the patient's performance, the nurse discussed this with the patient and pointed out what would be expected of her on the new system. Figure 5.7 shows an example of the record sheet which defined each target (e.g. be upstairs at 8.15 a.m.) along with a simple illustration of the target behaviour (see p. 97).

Graded Targets.   In Sally's case a small number of targets would be selected first. The goals would be made realistic by evaluating her ability on the baseline. If the initial goals are too high Sally will not achieve them, will receive few tokens and may become discouraged, if not even more disruptive. Alternatively, if the early goals are only a little more demanding than her present level she will earn many tokens, a lot of social approval and access to a large range of back-up reinforcers. Once her performance of one behaviour has reached the target level, the tokens may be reallocated to a new behaviour. Although she is losing reinforcement for one behaviour, adequate reinforcement will still be available to meet her needs, through this token transfer.

Accompanying Techniques. As in Mrs Smith's case the token economy could be used as the basis for a complex programme involving other techniques. The programme could include *social skills* training, where Sally could learn how to accept criticism, make a complaint appropriately, ask for favours, etc. Tokens could be used within the group and for homework assignments within the ward routine. A modified *stress inoculation* technique could be used to help Sally manage her anger and aggression. The nurse would try to help her detail the situations which made her angry, how she 'saw' these situations and how to respond differently. Sally might be encouraged to practise thinking 'No . . . I'm not going to start shouting . . . that just gets me into more trouble. I'm going for a walk.' In the same vein Sally might be helped to monitor some aspect of her programme, or even learn to give herself reinforcement. Once she has learned that she can be more 'effective' by following certain rules, she may become more willing to participate.

Treatment-for-groups: Everyday Living Skills Deficits

The Disturbed and Dependent Adolescent

Although Brian's problems are more fundamental, they may be no easier to resolve. Like Sally, he lacks important pro-social skills, like eating and dressing. He also shows little interest in appropriate social and recreational behaviour. Brian's problems are, however, more the result of lack of learning than lack of motivation. In common with other severely handicapped people it is all too easy to blame his behaviour on his 'condition'. Often the patient's diagnostic label results in less, rather than more, education and training being offered. Staff may believe that 'there is no point in trying to teach him anything: he'll never learn.' This negative viewpoint is often borne out in the manner of the self-fulfilling prophecy. He fails to learn from the standard education and training offered to him and is denied any special learning opportunity. Children like Brian often end up being cared for in hospital or at home, when they really need an intensive training programme to give them some degree of independence and control over their environment.

A vast body of evidence now exists to show that self-care and basic social skills can be acquired, even by severely mentally handicapped people. A range of behavioural approaches has also shown promising results in reducing some of the antisocial and self-destructive behaviour shown by such patients, whether this be of biological origin or a function of institutionalisation.[13]

Skills Training

Many of Brian's problems are the result of a lack of *appropriate* training. He has failed to acquire basic self-care and social skills by natural means. It will be necessary, therefore, to arrange more systematic training, where the same approach is applied in an intensive fashion. It may be necessary to arrange extra eating, dressing and toilet-use sessions, since existing routines may not allow enough time for adequate teaching. Before beginning any programme, the nurse must analyse each skill: developing a standard process for teaching the chain of behaviours which comprise the overall skill of eating, dressing, etc.

Systematic Approach. Once the major steps in the programme have been defined the nurse must identify all the stages between each step in the chain. Since a number of different nurses — and perhaps also Brian's mother — will be involved in the training, it is crucial that each person tackles the training in the same manner. The kind of prompts required and the procedure for fading out physical, gestural and verbal 'assistance' should also be defined clearly. The following extract from a typical dressing programme illustrates the stages in teaching a child to put on his pants (see Figure 9.2). Once stage (a) has been mastered the child progresses to (b) and so on.

(1) The nurse puts the pants over both feet and pulls them up to the child's hips. She then . . .

(a) Prompts (physically) child to grip pants . . . says 'Pull up your pants, Brian' . . . and assists child to pull up pants to waist.

(b) Points to pants . . . says 'Pull up your pants, Brian' and guides child's hands to hips . . . giving only slight physical prompt to pull up pants to waist.

(c) Points to pants and instructs child 'Pull up your pants, Brian' *only*.

(d) Gives instructions only.

Once the child has mastered 'pulling up from hips' the nurse moves on to the next stage.

(2) The nurse puts the pants over both feet and pulls them up to the child's *knees*. She then repeats (c) and (d) above.

(3) The nurse puts the pants over *feet* only: repeats (c) and (d).

Figure 9.2: Backward Chaining Steps in Dressing

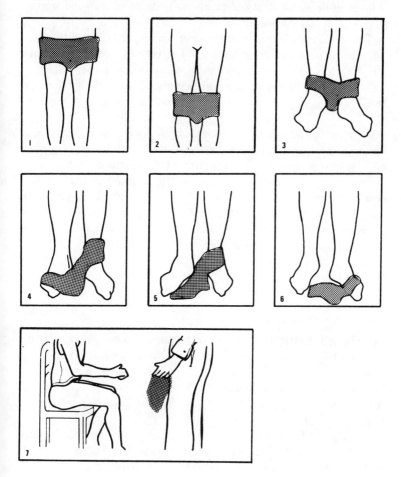

(4) The nurse puts the pants over *one* foot only, putting *toes* of other foot through the other leg. Instructs child to 'Put your other foot through, Brian' with accompanying gestures. She then repeats (c) and (d) above.

(5) The nurse puts left foot through and instructs child to 'Put your other foot through, Brian.' Repeats (c) and (d).

(6) The nurse puts pants over toes of left foot. Instructs child to 'Pull on your pants, Brian.' Instructs child to 'put the other leg through' and then repeats (c) and (d).

(7) Gives child the pants and tells him 'Put on your pants Brian.' If he is unsuccessful at any stage the nurse drops back to the previous stage and repeats the process.

This carefully scripted training programme gives nurses little room for creativity. However, it ensures that each person who operates the dressing programme uses the same approach as her colleagues and begins each day where Brian finished successfully the day before.

Motivation. Although the skills training is graded in difficulty, each step in the programme may be extremely difficult for Brian. The nurse must ensure that he is given plentiful reinforcement at each stage, to motivate him to continue. The details of the programme should include details of how much, of what kind of reinforcer, should be given. The criteria for witholding reinforcement (time-out) or withdrawing it (response-cost) should also be made explicit. Social approval should be given each time Brian follows an instruction: this might be accompanied by some preferred tangible reinforcer − such as a small piece of chocolate or a potato chip − which would be given continuously and then faded gradually on to a variable reinforcement schedule.

Eating Skills Training

Brian is able to use a spoon, but often prefers to eat with his fingers. He can become noisy and aggressive if forced to use his cutlery. The eating programme would attempt to improve his spoon use and to decrease his antisocial behaviour at the table (i.e. eating with his fingers, shouting, etc.). The programme would include the following stages.

(1) Brian's hand is placed firmly over the the spoon and the nurse instructs him as she guides the spoon through the scooping, lifting to mouth and returning to plate sequence. She praises Brian at the end of each small step. The major reinforcer will be the food on the plate, which should be selected from his reinforcer 'menu'.

(2)-(5) Brian's hand is released gradually further from his mouth (see Figure 9.3). This allows him to complete more and more of the eating behaviour independently. The nurse picks up the 'return-to-plate' prompt as soon as Brian has eaten the food from the spoon.

(6)-(10) The nurse transfers the scooping action to Brian's control by fading the physical prompts: initially the whole hand is guided, then the back of the hand only, then from the wrist, and finally from his arm and elbow.

Figure 9.3: Backward Chaining Steps in Eating

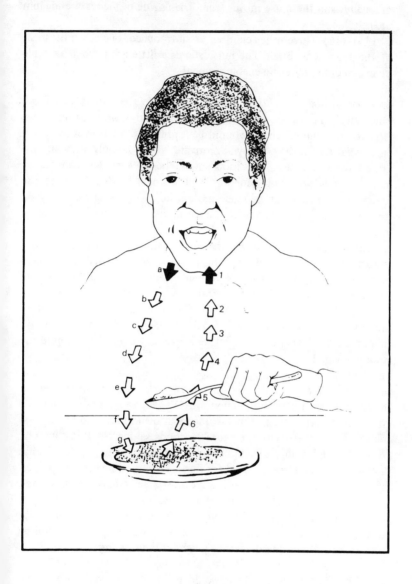

(11)-(13) The number of instructions and gestures is reduced gradually, and the nurse moves from Brian's side to the seat beside him at the table.

(14)-(16) Three other children are introduced, one at a time, to sit at the table with Brian. The nurse stands a little away from the table giving random praise and encouragement.

Materials.   Some attention should be paid to the cutlery and food, since this will play a major part in the acquisition of eating skills. The food, as noted above, should be a preferred 'reinforcer'. If Brian likes what he is eating, this will motivate him to comply with the new 'rules' for spoon use. The food should be of a stodgy consistency initially; this will help scooping and lifting. As Brian's spoon use improves, the food can be made more solid: progressing from a mash, to a fine mince, to small 'chunks', large chunks and finally, the ordinary meal itself.

The plate and spoon can be 'shaped' in a similar manner. In the early stages of training a child's feeding bowl, with one raised side to help scooping, can be used. This can be held steady on the table with a non-slip mat. As scooping becomes established, a flatter dish can be introduced and finally an ordinary plate. The spoon handle can be built up initially, with layers of tape, to make gripping easier. As Brian's grip improves, the layers can be removed gradually, until he can hold the spoon unaided.

Inappropriate Behaviour.   If Brian shows any unacceptable behaviour during the training session, action must be taken to 'punish' such behaviour. If he attempts to dip his fingers into the food, the nurse must remove the plate from the table for 30 seconds, saying 'No, Brian' sharply. Any food on his fingers should be wiped off immediately, before he has a chance to 'reinforce himself' for finger-feeding. If he becomes aggressive or noisy, the nurse should leave the table, taking the spoon and plate with her and returning in 30 seconds. If this is not successful, the time-out can be extended gradually, to 40, 50 seconds and so on. Since this procedure will prolong the mealtime, a warming plate should be used to keep Brian's meal warm throughout the training.

The Teaching Session.   Brian would progress from one stage of the programme to the next as soon as the nurse was satisfied that he was competent at that stage. The training will concentrate upon regular mealtimes but can be supplemented by additional spoon-use sessions, e.g. in mid-morning or afternoon. These extra sessions can be used to teach him to scoop cereal, potato chips or even sweets or drinks. Care should be taken to ensure that this does not upset his appetite at mealtimes. Alternatively, the size of his meals could be reduced, and several small meals given: e.g. six small meals per day, instead of three full meals. As other diners are introduced to the table, the nurse will attempt to shape up appropriate social-eating behaviour, punishing any stealing or throwing of food with a time-out procedure. Where other diners are involved it is more appropriate to remove Brian from the table, rather than taking the food away from him. He could be taken away to the side of the dining room where he can see the other diners eating and receiving the praise and attention of the nurse at the table. To operate this time-out procedure, another nurse will be needed to take Brian to and from the table.

Dressing Skills

The basic skills of spoon use are best established by using a backward chaining technique, as described above. The same technique will be used to establish basic dressing skills. Brian will be asked to *finish* the dressing action, in the manner described earlier, e.g. to pull up his pants from his hips to his waist. As progress is made, he will be asked to finish further and further back along the chain, until he can complete the whole action.

The whole dressing procedure is taught at each session. Brian would be prompted through putting on vest, pants, shirt, trousers, jersey, socks and shoes. Fastenings, such as buttons and zips, would be left to a separate programme. At each stage of the training, each garment would be at approximately the same level of difficulty. If Brian can pull up his pants from his ankles (mid-point in the chain) he will most likely be able to pull on his socks or jersey from the same stage.

The Teaching Session. If the nurse takes ten minutes to dress Brian, a backward chaining programme, such as the one described earlier, would take no more than 15 minutes. As the child is being asked only to *complete* the action, the nurse does most of the work in the early stages. This means that the dressing is completed at much the same pace; the nurse instructs the child as she goes through each action, asking him to do a little more each session. If Brian gets stuck at any stage the nurse returns to the previous stage, to help him succeed. As in the eating programme, Brian will be reinforced with social approval and some tangible reinforcement, each time he completes the stage of dressing. If time is available, a more intensive programme can be established, where Brian is taught to dress and undress repeatedly, each time doing a little more than previously. Learning by this approach may be faster since each stage of the training can be repeated several times, and there are no distractions, such as rushing to prepare for breakfast.

Materials. A shaping process can be used with Brian's clothes to make dressing and undressing easier. If slightly over-sized clothes are used, this makes it easier for Brian to perform the various arm and leg manoeuvres required. In the early stages of training a sticking fastener (such as Velcro) can be used as a substitute for zips. Over-sized buttons and buttonholes can be phased in gradually, and reduced in size over several weeks or months as Brian becomes more adept at fastening.

Response Cost. The reinforcers (such as peanuts or small pieces of chocolate) used in the dressing programme will be extra to the situation. These will be given for successful completion of each stage in the chain and will be witheld until Brian is successful. If he is unco-operative, a response-cost procedure can be used. The nurse would reprimand Brian and then would eat the reinforcer herself, showing Brian that it was lost forever.

Social Dressing. Once Brian has mastered the basic skills of dressing, through this individualised programme, he would be included in a small group, along the lines of the eating programme. Reinforcement would then be faded on to a variable schedule and would be supplemented by the vicarious reinforcement of Brian's peers within the group. The dressing programme would then progress from dressing routinely, to dressing for special occasions — such as visits from parents or trips to town — each of which will have their own built-in reinforcers.

Continence Training. Using the toilet appropriately is much more complicated than either of the two skills described above, and involves a number of discrete skills. The patient must be able to:

(1) recognise the 'need' to use the toilet;
(2) walk to the toilet;
(3) open the toilet door;
(4) undress;
(5) sit down or stand to urinate or defecate;
(6) wipe self as appropriate;

(7) dress and flush toilet;
(8) return to where he came from.

All these steps are essential for 'independent' toilet use. In the case of a very severely handicapped person, however, this may not be a realistic goal, and some of the steps may be removed from the programme. Backward chaining, once again, would be the most appropriate approach. In the early stages of training Brian would be taken to the toilet at the 'peak times' established from the assessment. The nurse would prompt him throughout each stage of undressing and sitting, etc., very little being required of Brian at this stage. For example:

Come on Brian, time for the toilet. (takes his hand and points to the door) This way Brian. (gestures towards door) Okay Brian, now open the door. (prompts him to grasp handle and turn, as necessary) Right then Brian, take your trousers down. (points and gestures, prompting physically as necessary) Okay Brian, now sit down. (prompts him to sit on seat) Good boy, well done.

Peak Times. Sitting on the toilet is advocated for males in the early stages of training, especially where the patient is doubly incontinent. Standing at the toilet or urinal can be taught at a later stage. Brian would be taken to the toilet at the 'peak time' and allowed to sit for no more than ten minutes. If he urinates or defecates this will be reinforced heavily. If he is unsuccessful, he is prompted to dress again and return to the ward, returning to the toilet at ten-minute intervals until he is successful. Once he has urinated or defecated he returns to the toilet at the next 'peak time' on the chart. Since one of Brian's problems is 'distractibility and hyperactivity' he may need to be trained to sit (e.g. on a chair) before beginning the toilet-training programme, by shaping longer and longer periods of sitting by use of tangible and social reinforcement.

The Rapid Method. An intensive toilet-training programme for day- and night-time enuresis, has been been developed by Foxx and Azrin.[14] By increasing the patient's fluid intake, the number of toilet visits — and learning opportunities — are increased. The patient usually visits the toilet every 30 minutes, after which he receives more fluids to maintain his need to urinate at regular intervals. This substantial increase in fluid intake should always be monitored by the patient's physician. As more 'hits' than 'misses' are recorded, the increased fluids are phased out and the patient visits the toilet only as necessary.

Dry Pants and Positive Practice. The 'rapid method' involves two specific targets: increasing appropriate toilet use and reducing incontinent episodes. The patient is reinforced not only for using the toilet, but also for 'being dry'. A procedure known as 'dry pants' training is incorporated in the skills training programme. The nurse checks the patient at regular intervals (e.g. every 30 minutes) and prompts him to feel his crotch as she asks, 'Are you dry, Brian?' If he is dry the nurse reinforces him with praise and an appropriate tangible reinforcer. If he is wet she says sharply, 'No, Brian, you are wet!' The child is then prompted, as necessary, to collect fresh clothing, to shower and change himself into dry underwear. Foxx and Azrin recommend that this 'overcorrection' procedure should include washing the soiled under-wear, mopping up any urine on the floor or seat, and a period of time spent going backwards and forwards to the toilet (positive practice). The whole process should be completed in a neutral manner: the nurse should not show any obvious emotion, as this may stimulate aggression in the patient, or may reinforce his incontinent behaviour.

Skills Training Summary

Where the patient shows major deficits of everyday living skills it may be necessary to arrange individualised treatment along the lines indic-ated. Once the patient has reached a satisfactory level, other patients can be introduced gradually, to form appropriate small-group pro-grammes. In these group exercises the programme will operate along the lines of the typical eating, grooming and personal hygiene routines of the ward. Not only will these small groups be cost-effective, but will provide an opportunity for vicarious learning and a simple foundation upon which to build basic interpersonal skills (e.g. table manners).

The key feature of the skills training approach described is the use of the task analysis.[15] Each skill is broken down into small steps: each of these are taught individually and then chained together with a backward chaining technique. A wide range of prompts is used initially. These are faded systematically — physical prompts first, then gestural and finally verbal — in order to ensure that the patient can take over control of the behaviour himself. Both social and tangible reinforcers are used in positive reinforcement and punishment techniques, in order to strengthen and weaken patterns of behaviour.

Anti-social Behaviour

Brian also shows two specific maladaptive behaviours: he is hyper-active and occasionally aggressive. Although a range of treatment methods is possible, we shall consider only two approaches here, one which is concerned with building up an incompatible behaviour and the other which us mainly aimed at reducing the maladaptive behaviour.

Attention Training. Staff suggest that Brian cannot sit still for very long, and that he pays no attention when they ask him to do even very simple things. The aims of any treatment programme would be to increase his 'attention to task' so that he can benefit from other train-ing programmes. The attention training programme would involve the following stages:

(1) The nurse places a chair in the centre of the floor and instructs the patient, 'Brian . . . come and sit down.' She then guides him to the seat, her left hand over his left arm and the palm of her right hand in his back. She then repeats the instruction 'sit down Brian' when they reach the chair, placing her hands on his shoulders and pressing him gently downwards to the chair. As soon as he 'sits' she praises him generously and gives him a preferred reinforcer. She then stands in front of him and reinforces him for sitting, at ten second intervals, for two or three minutes. During this time the nurse shapes up eye-contact by prompting the patient to 'look at me, Brian' using the reinforcer to catch his attention and giving this to him as soon as eye-contact is made. (See Figure 9.4.) She now takes a step backwards and puts out her hand, prompting the patient to 'come here, Brian', reinforcing him as soon as he steps towards her.

(2)-(5) The nurse repeats the steps described above, but fades her prompts gradually and delays reinforcement until it is given at (apparently) random intervals during the period of sitting. She con-tinues to praise him liberally throughout the whole sequence.

(6) The nurse prompts Brian to sit down and then takes up a position a few feet away from the chair. She continues to reinforce him for eye-contact on a variable schedule, giving social approval each time he looks at her on request. If he rises from the seat she prompts him to sit down again, but does not reinforce him for doing so.

(7)-(10) The nurse takes up positions further and further from the chair, asking Brian to walk to the seat, sit down and walk across the room to her, independently. Once this sitting on command is

Figure 9.4: Shaping Eye-contact

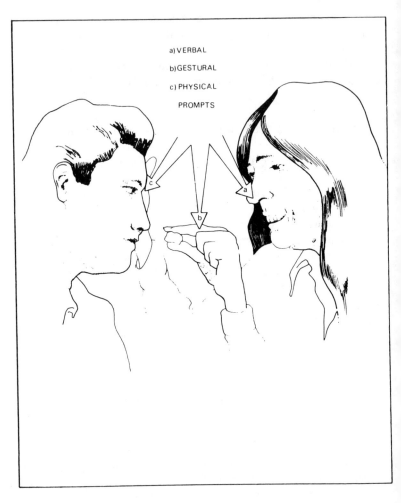

established, the skill is 'generalised' to other parts of the ward, where Brian is prompted to sit down and look at books, pick up blocks, etc., using the same prompting and reinforcement procedure.

Overcorrection. Brian's aggressive and stereotypic behaviour (e.g. spinning and rocking) could be tackled by Foxx and Azrin's overcorrection methods.[16] There are two major procedures. *Positive practice* is generally applied to stereotypic behaviours and is similar to the habit reversal technique described in Chapter 7. The patient is required to practise a more appropriate form of the relevant behaviour. Stereotypes are self-reinforcing and therefore self-perpetuating. By requiring him to practise an incompatible behaviour – such as standing still instead of spinning – the stereotyped action is extinguished (i.e. self-reinforcement is stopped) *and* punished (by the enforced positive practice). Each time Brian begins spinning or rocking, the nurse would shout 'No', take hold of his arms and hold them at his side, bringing him to a standstill. She holds him in this position for one minute and then prompts him to sit down again. The amount of strong physical prompting can be reduced as Brian becomes less resistive and he begins to stop spinning and rocking on request.

In *restitution* the patient is required to correct the consequences of his disruptive actions. If Brian knocks over chairs or toys while spinning, he would be prompted to go back and 'correct' the situation by setting chairs and tables upright and putting toys back in their place. This procedure is used in continence training where the patient has to mop up urine or wash his soiled underwear.

Overcorrection and Punishment. The overcorrection technique consists of a number of factors including extinction, time-out from reinforcement, response prevention, physical restraint, prompting, reinforcement of competing responses and changes in the patient's social environment. It is difficult to determine which combination of these factors is responsible for the success of overcorrection. Without doubt this is a punishment technique: it reduces behaviour and is unpleasant as far as the patient is concerned. However, this technique may be more acceptable to nurses than other punishment methods, and may be more effective with disruptive and stereotyped behaviour than the use of time-out or differential reinforcement methods. The use of 'forcible' prompting and physical restraint may, however, cause some ethical hackles to rise. Although it can be argued that overcorrection is preferable to sedation or seclusion, it involves the physical manipulation of the patient and, if not strictly controlled and supervised, could lead to accidental injury.

The two packages described are aimed at reducing socially disruptive behaviour. One approach tries to increase adaptive behaviour which is mutually exclusive to the problem, whilst the other concentrates upon reducing the problem more directly. Both methods would then be applied, initially, within the context of an individual programme; later, they would be used in the patient's social situation, to aid generalisation.

The ultimate aim of the programme would be to give Brian the opportunity to participate in groups – in the playroom, dining room or toilet area – where his training could be supplemented by some vicarious learning, through the experience of his peer group.

Group Therapy: A Summary

In this chapter we have discussed the use of standardised 'packages' in the treatment of a wide range of social behaviour problems. These have been presented as illustrations of *possible* solutions, and should not be interpreted as the only way by which these problems could be resolved. In each illustration, treatment is geared towards the individual. The programme can, however, be applied as part of the processes of group interaction (treatment *through* groups), in the patient's everyday social setting (treatment *in* groups) or as a preparation for participation in low-level social activities (treatment *for* groups). Each package embraces a basic range of behavioural techniques which can be complemented by other methods where appropriate.

A patient like Mrs Smith may have a central problem, such as assertion deficit, which if resolved may have many positive spin-offs, giving her the confidence to start resolving other problems of living independently. The group setting acts as the medium for treatment; peer group support, modelling and vicarious reinforcement are available here, where they would be missing from individual therapy. In this kind of group setting the nurse has an opportunity to strengthen the patient's independence, by sharing her attention evenly amongst the group members and using the group to generate solutions to the patient's problems.

Some aspects of Sally's antisocial behaviour could be called 'learned'. Explosive outbursts, apathy or disinhibited behaviour are typical of institutionalised patients. These problems are compounded by features of her organic pathology (such as her memory defect). The behavioural treatment programme described is not concerned to treat a patient with Korsakoff's psychosis. However, the resocialisation programme must take account of her disabilities and must acknowledge that her capacity for relearning may be severely impaired. The token economy format, as illustrated, can be adapted to suit the patient, without disrupting the existing social structure of her life on the ward. For the truly chronic patient, like Sally, such an approach may be one of the best ways of ensuring that she maintains what independence and dignity she has left.

Brian's social behaviour problems are equally complex. His lack of social and self-care skills could be attributed to his severe mental defect. Although he is intellectually impaired and may have brain damage, this is not an adequate explanation of his lack of social behaviour. Brian's treatment programme aims to give him some basic social skills through intensive individual therapy, after which he may benefit from participation in group activities. All three of our 'patients' are social animals: the nurse has a prime responsibility for maintaining, or giving, the patient the skills needed to function better within his or her own social group.

Notes

1. Lazarus, A.A. 'Group therapy of phobic disorders by systematic desensitisation', *Journal of Abnormal and Social Psychology*, vol. 63 (1961), pp. 505–10.

2. For a brief review of this research, see: Sherman, R.A. *Behaviour Modification: Theory and Practice* (Monterey, California, Brooks/Cole, 1973), pp. 62–4.

3. Kazdin, A.E. *The Token Economy* (New York, Plenum Press, 1977).

4. Salter, A. *Conditioned Reflex Therapy* (New York, Creative Age, 1949).

5. Wolpe, J. 'The instigation of assertive behaviour. Transcripts from two cases', *Journal of Behaviour Therapy and Experimental Psychiatry*, vol. 1 (1970), pp. 145–51.

6. Trower, P., Bryant, B. and Argyle, M. *Social Skills and Mental Health* (London, Methuen, 1978).

7. Goldstein, A.P. Sprafkin, R.P. and Gershaw, N.J. *Skill Training for Community Living: Applying Structured Learning Therapy* (New York, Pergamon Press, 1976).

8. Liberman, R.P., King, L.W., DeRisi, W.J. and McCann, M. *Personal Effectiveness: Guiding People to Assert Themselves and Improve their Social Skills* (Champaign, Illinois, Research Press, 1975).

9. Ayllon, T. and Azrin, N.H. *The Token Economy: A Motivational System for Therapy and Rehabilitation* (New York, Appleton Century Crofts, 1968).

10. Barker, P., Docherty, P., Hird, J. and Hunter, M.H. 'Living and learning: a nurse-administered token economy programme involving mentally handicapped schoolboys', *International Journal of Nursing Studies*, vol. 15 (1978), pp. 91–102.

11. McFadden, H. 'Behavioural treatment of a patient with Korsakoff's psychosis', *CCNS Course Reports* (unpublished report, Royal Dundee Liff Hospital, 1979).

12. Portues, C. 'The use of self-monitoring with a hospitalised psychotic patient', *CCNS Course Reports* (unpublished report, Royal Dundee Liff Hospital, 1981).

13. For a review of treatment approaches to self-injury, see: Rapoff, M.A., Altman, K. and Christopherson, E.R. 'Suppression of self-injurious behaviour: determining the least restrictive alternative', *Journal of Mental Deficiency Research*, vol. 24 (1980), pp. 37–46

14. Azrin, N.H. and Foxx, R.M. 'A rapid method of toilet training the institutionally retarded', *Journal of Applied Behaviour Analysis*, vol. 4 (1971), pp. 89-99.

15. For detailed illustrations of training programmes based upon task analysis, see: Watson, L.S. *How to Use Behaviour Modification with Mentally Retarded and Autistic Children* (Columbus, Ohio, Behaviour Modification Technology, 1972).

16. Foxx, R.M. and Azrin, N.H. 'The elimination of autistic self-stimulatory behaviour by overcorrection', *Journal of Applied Behaviour Analysis*, vol. 6 (1973), pp. 1-14.

10 THE NURSE AS THERAPIST

> 'Not to get emotionally involved' is one of the chief worries
> of large-city people. This state of affairs, not quite avoidable
> for any of us, already bears the stamp of inhumanity.
> — Konrad Lorenz

Helping the Patient

Nursing Roles

Although the behavioural approach can be effective with a wide range
of problems of living, many patients are still denied therapy, due largely
to a shortage of appropriately trained 'therapists'. Over the last decade
many authors have documented the increasing contribution made by
nurses to a variety of behavioural programmes.[1-3] Indeed, it has been
argued that nursing may be the only health-care profession with sufficient numbers to ensure that the demand for behaviour therapy is met,
on a scale commensurate with its demonstrated effectiveness.[4,5]

The concept of nurse behaviour therapist is, however, by no means
fully implemented or even accepted. There is, however, general agreement that nurses can extend their therapeutic skills without sacrificing
too much of their traditional caring role.[6] Nurses can now train to
work as specialists in the community, receiving referrals direct from
family doctors and assuming the central therapeutic role of case
manager.[7] In hospitals a different role model is required. Some nurses
work as full-time 'consultants', advising other nurses on the management of patients, planning treatment programmes and conducting
research. Other nurses incorporate aspects of the behavioural approach
into routine care programmes or to augment patient management
systems. If this trend continues nursing will benefit by acquiring the
therapeutic skills and research orientation of the behavioural approach
which, in turn, will become available to a much wider audience.[8]

The Care-giver as Change-agent. The nurse clearly has a potential role
as a behaviour therapist, whether this is within the traditional role
model or in a more specialist capacity. Although nurses have operated
as therapists in many different clinical settings in the past (e.g. the
therapeutic community) the concept of the nurse as a change-agent
is of more recent origin. The association between nurses and behaviour

therapy is probably no more than twenty years old. In one of the earliest projects involving nurses, Ayllon and Michael[9] described the treatment of a range of psychotic and institutionalised behaviours: persistent entering the nursing station, hoarding, 'crazy talk', eating problems and aggressive behaviour. The programme was designed and supervised by a psychologist, but was carried out by nurses as part of their routine care. Although it has been argued that these problems were not the most serious to be met within a typical psychiatric setting, they were (and still are) typical of the behaviour problems which are highly resistant to traditional treatment methods and with which nurses cope daily, often unaided. Ayllon and Michael's study, which involved modifying the nurses' interactions with their patients, inspired many others to consider the nurse's role as change-agent as well as care-giver.

In recent years the nurse's role as dispenser of 'tender, loving care' has met with much criticism, none more damning than the findings of a study by Gelfand and her colleagues.[10] This showed that nurses tended to ignore patients when they showed desirable, or 'non-psychotic', behaviour. Instead they gave intermittent reinforcement to 'sick' or manifestly psychotic behaviour. The nurses involved in the study took the view that their patients were crippled by negative self-evaluations. As a result, they needed warmth and sympathy to re-establish their self-esteem. The authors noted that this viewpoint was advocated by some standard nursing textbooks. In the case of a mute patient nurses were advised to handle him by 'sitting by him for long periods and doing little things like combing his hair or getting him a drink'.[11] This orientation led, in the authors' view, to the unintentional reinforcement of 'sick' behaviour, since only very withdrawn patients were afforded such intimate and specialised attention. This caring orientation is evident in nurses' attitudes to other patient groups. Although nurses are beginning to embrace a training or educational model in mental handicap care, the traditional approach in this field has been supportive and custodial. Where patients' problems are seen as intractable, 'total care' is often given; this usually means attending to diet, clothing and hygiene, rather than training or education. Ironically, this humanitarian ethos can produce side-effects. It has been shown, for example, that handicapped people who live in a state of total dependence are more likely to show disturbed behaviour of an aggressive, destructive or self-mutilative nature. Although such extreme behaviour occurs as a by-product of the patient's interaction with a severely restricted environment, it is often associated, misguidedly, with the condition of mental handicap itself. Where nurses view behaviour as a natural consequence of the patient's clinical condition, they are unlikely to take consistent action to change such behaviour.

Studies, such as those referred to above, have shown that nurses can act as disabling agencies, through their attempts to provide total care for the patient. It would appear that some, though clearly not all, aspects of the patient's behaviour are manufactured and maintained by the care system, rather than determined by nature.

The Development of Psychiatric Nursing. The caring orientation of nurses did not develop by accident. Nurses began as the custodians of all classes of insane people, both mentally ill and handicapped, in the asylums of the early nineteenth century. Lunacy was seen as mainly of moral or physical origin. Since physicians were the only interested parties, the solution to the lunacy problem involved, primarily, a search for the physical origins of mental disorder. This search was reinforced by Noguchi's discovery of the syphilitic origins of general paralysis of the insane, the detection of the chromosomal abnormalities of mongolism, and later by the identification of other variants of mental defect of genetic or traumatic origin. Although organic causes for the rest of the 'mental illnesses' failed to materialise, and in spite of Seguin's pioneering success in the education of 'idiots', physical care and treatment remained the central model of care provision. The development of psychological theories of mental disorder did little to change the nurse's role, although ultimately these were to have a radical effect upon society's view of mental illness. Instead, the development of psychotropic drugs in the 1950s again enhanced the reputation of the medical model of care and gave nurses a more satisfactory means of controlling severely disturbed patients. Aspects of the nurse's role as the doctor's handmaiden, holding the keys to the cells and chains of the madhouse, still persist 150 years later, as she guards the keys to the ward and the drug cabinet.

General nursing, with its emphasis upon the care of the sick and dying, has always been held in high regard by society at large. It was not surprising that the emphasis upon general nursing principles and practice should be increased when general nurses assumed overall responsibility for the training of nurses in the mental field. More than twenty years were to pass before the benefits of such an overtly medical approach to the mentally ill and handicapped was questioned. By the end of the 1970s, however, nurses in mental handicap were expressing severe disenchantment with their training and psychiatric nurses argued that the general nursing orientation of their training militated against an effective therapeutic role.[12] At the beginning of the 1980s many nurses argue that a serious analysis of nursing, *by nurses themselves*, will be necessary not only to meet the needs of the patient, but also to ensure the future of the profession.[13]

The Needs of the Patient. If nurses are dissatisfied with their subordinate role as the doctor's handmaiden, what do they see as a viable alternative? Nursing has been defined, in general, as an activity in which the nurse *helps* the patient to perform those activities which he would perform unaided had he the necessary strength, will or knowledge. Nurses often share the patient's everyday experience, spending more time with him than any other health-care professional. Taken together, the *time* nurses invest upon *everyday living skills* signifies at least one facet of the uniqueness of nursing. This has led to the description of nursing as a 'situational activity, centred upon goals for living, rather than a disease/illness concept alone'.[14] Nursing is concerned with meeting human needs, whether they are of physical, emotional, intellectual or social origin. This 'patient-centred', rather than task-oriented, approach is aimed at raising the patient's potential for independent living.

Viewed from this angle most forms of nursing can be called learning situations, where the nurse teaches the patient how to monitor his 'condition' or how to adapt his lifestyle to suit the significant factors of his biological or social situation. Although nurses help doctors to diagnose and treat the patient, their distinctive role lies in helping the patient deal with the change in the relationship with himself, which has been caused by his mental illness or handicap. She is concerned primarily to help him overcome his problems of living. In order to achieve this goal nursing must be built around the particular, perhaps idiosyncratic, features of the person called 'patient'. Only by viewing the patient as a person can appropriate and effective care be given. Nurses cannot afford to view the patient as though he existed in a vacuum. They must take into account those aspects of his social and physical environment, as well as his biological make-up, which significantly affect his problems of living. As Gelfand demonstrated, the goal of nursing will only be realised if nurses can transform their interactions with patients into helping, rather than hindering, relationships.

If nurses are to meet the needs of their patients on a comprehensive scale, they must embrace a therapeutic, as well as caring, philosophy. If we use the definitions of nursing which are given above as a guideline, the terms therapeutic and caring become synonymous. Although a small proportion of patients (such as the terminally ill) are unlikely to regain even minimal degrees of independence, overall, nursing is concerned with establishing or restoring the patient's dignity and self-respect through greater independence. Even where truly chronic patients are concerned nurses must attempt to maintain their status as independent human beings, rather than fostering (albeit unwittingly) a dependent invalid. Although the principle of this therapeutic-caring approach has been established, its practice has, as yet, to be fully documented.

The Nursing Process

Nurses have, traditionally, been subject to medical authority and supervision. As a result, sociologists view nursing as merely a semi-professional sector, rather than a fully-fledged profession. Although many nurses work independent of any medical direction, their activity tends to be ill-defined, unresearched and manifestly unscientific in character. Where nurses *assume* authority in the clinical setting, they may have little to fall back on if required to justify this.[15] The unprofessionalism of nursing is not confined to mental health. Nursing care plans in general are still often based upon inadequate assessment, may fail to specify the contribution of different grades of staff and may concentrate upon the nurse's role as a medical support service.[16] However, nurses are now trying to break away from their task-oriented and supportive role in favour of the client-centred model which (theorists have claimed for many years) personifies the very essence of nursing. Nurses are trying to delineate a process of nursing which will identify the specialist body of skill and knowledge which will distinguish nursing from other health-care professions.

The 'nursing process' is the term which has been used to describe the principles of clinical management drawn from a study of the needs of the individual patient.[17] This involves the identification of the patient's needs (assessment), the selection and implementation of an appropriate course of action (planning and intervention) and the evaluation of whether or not the need has been met.

The Behavioural Approach. The nursing process is mirrored, with little distortion, in the methodology of behaviour therapy (see Chapter 1). Both approaches view the patient as a person with a performance problem, both study him against the backdrop of his everyday experience, rather than in isolation, and both devise a therapeutic programme based upon these assessment data which is then evaluated carefully.

Although this nursing process may help us monitor nurse–patient interaction, it gives little guidance as to the exact nature of that inter-action. How will the nurse fulfill the patient's needs? What will she do to help him? Nurses may continue, for the foreseeable future, to seek advice from other disciplines and sciences, to answer this question. For instance, once a nurse has identified that a patient is hungry she must turn to dietetics for advice upon what to offer him to eat, to biology for an understanding of how he will react to the food and to medical science for a remedy when problems are encountered (e.g. in absorbing certain nutrients). She may also turn to psychology for advice about how best to structure a comfortable dining situation, or to sociology or anthropology for an understanding of attitudes to food and eating, expressed by different cultures or sub-cultures. We should remember, therefore, that we can *use* the skills and knowledge of other sciences without losing our nursing identity. We do not need to be a cartographer to read a road map, or an electrician to mend a fuse. Similarly, we do not need to be a psychologist to practise behaviour therapy. Our skill as a therapist will, however, be influenced by the training given: this principle applies, of course, to any aspect of the nurse's work. Nurses have always expressed a number of sciences – notably biological science – in their attempts to meet the needs of the patient. Perhaps the ability to select, co-ordinate and present, the skills and knowledge of an *appropriate* science is the hallmark of a truly helpful nurse.

Reluctance to Change.   Many of the needs of psychiatric and mental handicap patients are of a psycho-social character. As a result, the behavioural approach may have an important role as an 'appropriate scientific input'. If nurses ignore the behavioural approach, with many problems of living they will soon exhaust the range of 'scientific' possibilities open to them. If, for instance, the patient is incontinent the nurse may arrange for a medical examination to isolate any genito-urinary problems. If these are ruled out she may only have regular toiletting, restriction of fluids and incontinence pads as available options to raise the patient's potential for 'not wetting the floor'. It would be naive in the extreme to assume that behaviour therapy can provide an answer to every conceivable problem of living. How-ever, a range of well-researched and carefully packaged interventions are available, the value of which should not be underestimated. The approach also provides a framework for designing and evaluating new treatment or training programmes. Although numerous studies have identified nurses' weaknesses in dealing with certain problems, and have offered alternatives, some nurses are reluctant to adopt a behavioural orientation. This may be due to a misconception as to the exact nature of the behavioural model. In many circles behaviourism is associated only with Pavlovian conditioning experiments or some of the cruder and more restrictive examples of operant conditioning. Apart from any ethical considerations which they invoke these animal-based models appear to be alien to the humanitarian ethos of nursing. Sadly, this distorted perspective is often amplified by writers who wish to score a point for some competing model of care or treatment.[18]

As we have argued throughout this book, the behavioural approach has no ethical code of its own. It can be used by sinner and saint alike. We cannot criticise behaviour therapy, only those who use it unwisely or recklessly. If we accept the views expressed by observers of the nursing scene, or eminent nurses themselves, then we must accept that nursing is all about changing patient behaviour, either intentionally or unwittingly. It does this in the name of rehabilitation, with liberal sprinklings of care and compassion. If nurses cannot restore the patient to something like his former, effective self, they will, at least, try to maintain his dignity and self-respect, even at the height of his distress or as his life draws to a close. Behavioural technology can offer no assurance to achieve these ends. Like other technologies it is a mere tool which, in the right hands, can be wielded to advantage, but which may be useless or dangerous in the hands of the incompetent. Although the nurse's role as a change-agent may be natural and established, it has yet to achieve a truly professional status. Behaviour therapy, with its reservoir of skills and knowledge, could help nurses to do well, what they already do unwittingly or at times with only limited success.

Models of Practice

From a review of the literature LeBow[19] identified three basic role models for nurses involved in behaviour therapy. They may be concerned with (1) the delivery of care direct to the patient, (2) the planning of care programmes and (3) the teaching of others about the use of behavioural methods. In the role of teacher, the nurse may teach other nurses, other professionals, the patient's family or the patient himself. In the typical nursing situation four distinct roles emerge: these are the practical outcome of the models described by LeBow. Nurses may act as the *presenters* of the programme, or as the overall *co-ordinators* of the patients' care. In other settings some nurses may act as independent, and highly skilled, *practitioners*, dealing mainly with individual patients. In a very small number of situations nurses may act as *consultants* to other nurses, dispensing advice, planning treatment programmes, arranging and conducting educational and research programmes. The roles of presenter and co-ordinator are the most common and therefore the most important for main-stream nursing. We shall discuss each of these roles in turn, alluding only briefly to the more specialist roles.

The Presenter

In the majority of psychiatric and mental handicap hospitals the staff who spend most time with the patient are either unqualified nursing 'aides' or nursing students. The situation in the community is quite different. Most community-based nurses have received some post-basic training in community work or will have a depth of practical experience. Although these nurses 'present' care to the patient, they operate primarily within the 'practitioner' role model (see below).

Most nurses who present behavioural programmes will have only minimal involvement in their planning. The nurses described in Ayllon and Michael's study operated at this level, with a psychologist acting as planner and supervisor. These nurses act mainly as technicians, a title which many nurses may resent. However, the situation in a behavioural programme would appear to be no different from the delivery of other nursing procedures. The senior nurse on the ward is responsible for the actions of her staff. As a result, she delegates only those activities which she is confident that the nurses can carry out competently. Even then some procedures may only be conducted under the supervision of a suitably qualified person, the junior nurse acting purely in a technical capacity.

The unique feature of the presenter is her proximity to the patient. The senior nurse, the nursing consultant, or some other professional, such as a psychologist, may have the all-important skills and knowledge necessary to change the patient's behaviour. However, the presenter, by virtue of her direct and regular contact with the patient, may be the best medium for the delivery of these skills. She may be the person best placed to change the patient's behaviour.

Targets. Junior nurses may act as programme presenters in a wide variety of settings with diverse problems. In an acute psychiatric ward nurses, with no previous experience of behaviour therapy, carried out a successful treatment of a patient with a two-year history of obssessive-compulsive avoidance behaviour and a severe germ phobia.[20] Working under the supervision of a visiting psychologist, these nurses collected the baseline data and applied a number of treatment methods when the patient performed obsessive rituals during showering, hand-washing and using the toilet. They also operated a more general treatment programme for her germ contamination phobia.

Numerous reports have discussed the nurse's role as therapist with long-stay psychiatric patients. Working with individuals, nurses carried out treatments which were designed by a psychologist, to reinstate speech in mute patients.[21] Working within 15-minute sessions, the nurse showed the patient pictures and asked him a series of standardised questions, ending the session with more open-ended questions of a more conversational nature. A range of prompting and reinforcement procedures were used to establish more coherent replies to questions about the patient and his surroundings. Programmes with groups of patients have concentrated upon the restoration of self-care and domestic skills, often using the token economy.[22] These programmes usually incorporate a range of prompting, shaping, modelling and reinforcement procedures, with or without an in-built punishment system, such as response-cost.

In mental handicap settings nurses with very limited experience have presented training programmes in basic care (e.g. feeding) or in the treatment of disturbed behaviour (e.g. regurgitation and faecal smearing).[23] Although these programmes are often straightforward in the early stages, when, for example, reinforcement schedules or some form of generalisation is introduced, they may become much more complex. Where the nurse is required to work for long periods in close proximity to very difficult patients, this may prove to be very demanding. In such situations careful staff selection and training may be needed in the early stages, followed by sustained 'emotional support' from senior nurses or other interested professionals.

Training. Although the presenter is required only to act as a technician, this does not mean that her role is always a simple one. In the examples quoted above the nurses required some personal qualities, as well as professional skills, to guarantee the success of the programme. These nurses do not simply carry out orders, but are required to report on progress, identify problems, whether actual or potential, and to administer the behavioural prescription with the skill and consistency required. To fulfil these requirements nurses must either be experienced, or willing to undergo some form of training.

A range of possibilities exists for training junior nurses in behavioural methods. Teaching of a practical nature can be offered on the ward by the senior nurse or some visiting consultant. Simple training in behavioural principles can be given in the form of lectures and seminars backed up by a regular test of the nurse's knowledge. In view of the overtly 'clinical' nature of the presenter's work, training should always be geared to the acquisition of practical skills first and academic knowledge last. If the ward or unit intends to develop the behavioural approach along more permanent lines, then more formal training opportunities must be offered. To date most of these in-service training exercises have concentrated upon the work with the more severely handicapped[24] and the rehabilitation of long-stay psychiatric patients.[25]

Staff Management.   The provision of training and a realistic treatment 'prescription' are not always sufficient to ensure that the programme is delivered successfully. The presenters must also be managed carefully to ensure that their initial enthusiasm does not dissipate, or that they are not upset by problems or failures. (Chapter 6 discusses the management of the nursing team in more general terms.) Many authors have suggested that junior staff need specific incentives — such as praise, the choice of shifts or holidays — to guarantee their co-operation. Some studies have shown that the presenters may need systematic encouragement from the programme 'consultants' in order to run the programme independently. In one study[26] nurses were given training during the planning stage and were then motivated through 'inspirational group meetings'. However, when they were left to run the programmes as part of their daily routine, their performance was most erratic. When the 'consultant' (a psychologist) telephoned the ward each day — to give praise for having run the programme or reminding the nurses to do so — this led to the nurses carrying out the programme each and every day thereafter. Although we might expect the senior nurse on the ward to ensure that any essential care or treatment is given we must be aware that some nurses are not sufficiently confident of their own abilities, or sufficiently self-motivated, to operate independently. In these situations support and encouragement may be needed from significant outsiders, especially when the programme is in its infancy.

The Co-ordinator

As we have noted, the presenter needs someone to provide in-service training, to supervise her work with the patient and to link with the designer of the programme. These co-ordinating functions are, typically, the responsibility of the senior nurse on the ward, the charge nurse or her deputy. In some cases this nurse may have received only limited training in behaviour therapy. In most situations, however, the advantages of a fully qualified nurse behaviour therapist acting as co-ordinator should be obvious.

The co-ordinator is responsible for adapting the nursing policy to ensure that all care and treatment programmes operate efficiently. She must co-ordinate this with other 'non-behavioural' inputs. Even within the tightest behavioural programme the patient still requires to be fed, clothed and perhaps given medication. He also needs a stimulating and comfortable environment. Although she may not supply all of these things, the co-ordinator must arrange (and take responsibility) for their delivery.

The co-ordinator is usually responsible for the selection and training of the staff who will be in face-to-face contact with the patient. Not all nurses are equipped, by personality or training, for the role of programme presenter. The co-ordinator must select only those nurses who she thinks have the necessary aptitude, and then must arrange some scheme of on-the-job training to give them the necessary skills and knowledge to run the programme. The co-ordinator will also be more involved in planning the programme than the presenters. Where she is a trained nurse therapist she may undertake this task independently. In other situations she may seek the assistance of other nurses or a psychologist for aspects of the planning or teaching role. Some authors believe that this nurse should be a clinical nurse specialist,[27] possessing a high degree of skill and knowledge related to the specific patient population concerned. Where such a nurse exists she may make 'consultants', such as those described by Ayllon and Michael, completely redundant.

Targets. Where a well-qualified co-ordinator is available more complex forms of treatment are possible. In acute psychiatric settings nurses have co-ordinated hospital teams in the treatment of very difficult problems such as anorexia nervosa.[28] In this situation the nurse ensured that the work of the psychiatrist, pharmacist, dietician and other nurses was suitably co-ordinated in addition to supervising the delivery of the behavioural programme.

In work with psychotic patients again the emphasis has been upon rehabilitation, with self-care and social skills taking priority. Where nurses are available on the ward to co-ordinate the treatment programme, this may be less rigid than those examples previously mentioned and is more likely to be self-maintaining.[29] In mental handicap settings more intensive forms of therapy can be presented, where a range of self-care deficits and maladaptive behaviours are treated within the one patient, rather than single problems.

Training. Schemes of training of a specialised nature are now becoming established, to equip nurses for this co-ordinating role. These programmes emphasise the acquisition of in-depth knowledge about assessment and treatment methods, often related to one patient population.[30] The training also emphasises the development of high-level skills in the use of these principles. In addition, nurses are required to learn the benefits of searching the literature — to identify the most appropriate and up-to-date methods — and are given an introduction to behavioural research methods. Although these nurses may work directly with patients, their distinctive role is the transmission of skills and knowledge to other nurses through in-service training or clinical modelling.

The Specialist Nurses

Opportunities have developed within the last decade for nurses to operate in a more specialised role as 'nurse behaviour therapist'. Although the career structure is still at an early stage of development, the clinical precedent of nurses acting as highly-skilled clinicians, or as consultants to other nurses, has already been established. Although the number of nurses in these positions is unlikely to be large, they are destined to occupy senior positions in an expanding clinical career structure. Until recently nurses working directly with patients had limited career prospects. If they wished to progress beyond the charge nurse/ward sister grade, they were required to leave the clinical setting in favour of employment as a nurse manager or nurse tutor. With the development of nurse practitioners and nurse consultants the potential for nurses to gain in status and recompense has increased, without requiring them to leave the clinical field.

The Practitioner. In a number of clinical settings it may be necessary to have a central therapist who is highly skilled and in a position to present the treatment programme. Although it is difficult to distinguish the simple from the complex case, it is apparent that some patients, as in the examples quoted, respond to therapy even when applied by nurses with limited skills and experience. However, in some settings a more skilled presenter will be required: e.g. in the community the practitioner may treat the patient in his own home or operate from a specialised out-patient clinic. This nurse may also work with selected patients who have been admitted to hospital, usually as short-term cases.

The role of the practitioner is more autonomous than that of the other two groups mentioned. Patients will be referred directly to her, either from a psychiatric service or from a general practitioner or health centre. The nurse will assess the patient, devise a treatment plan and carry this out independently, asking for assistance only when the treatment situation demands it − e.g. asking for a co-therapist in a group treatment programme. The role of these nurses and the nature of their caseload has been well described in the literature.[31]

Most nurse practitioners work with acute psychiatric patients, such as phobics, obsessionals, sexual and marital problems. They may also run groups for patients with problems which may benefit from exposure in groups, problems such as alcoholism, social anxieties or obesity. With some patients they may direct their efforts at establishing peer-group support through a self-help group, as in agoraphobia. Although this role is much less well publicised, practitioners are fulfilling an active role in providing individualised treatment to residents in hostels for the mentally ill, severely disturbed mentally handicapped children, and in day-care facilities for psychotic patients.

The Consultant. The nurse consultant in behaviour therapy is distinguished by her publicised position as 'on-call' adviser to her nursing colleagues. This nurse usually has a roving commission, working across a number of units, or even hospitals, dispensing information and advice, planning specialised treatment or training programmes and arranging educational programmes for different grades of staff. As a nurse she is likely to have an advantage over other 'consultants', such as psychologists, who often find that professional boundaries restrict them in their role as the overall director of the behavioural programme.

The nurse consultant usually carries a caseload of patients and devotes a proportion of her time to a practitioner role. This ensures that she maintains contact with the reality of the clinical situation and acts as an appropriate model to all the clinical nurses operating at the levels of responsibility below her. She is likely also to carry some managerial responsibilities: she may direct a small team of practitioners working in the community or co-ordinators working in designated behavioural wards in hospital. Some of her time will be spent negotiating for funds for staffing and in the administration of routine clinical as well as research programmes. She is also likely to be the key liaison figure linking the nurses who deliver therapy with other 'consultants' in the health-care team.

In addition to clinical, educational and administrative roles, this nurse is likely to be involved deeply in research. Nursing research in psychiatry is, as yet, in its infancy; most studies have concentrated upon role models, education or staffing policies. Comparatively few studies have looked at what nurses actually do for their patients. The nurse specialist claims to be helping the patient with his 'problems of living' and behaviour therapy claims to be based upon 'the scientific method'. This pairing would suggest that nurse-behaviour-therapy is an area ripe for clinical research. The nurse consultant, with her sophisticated knowledge and greater degree of freedom than her other senior nursing colleagues, may be the person best placed to set up and direct such research.

Therapeutic Skills

Nurses are unlikely to resolve the patient's problems of living by exercising technical skills alone. The success of behaviour therapy depends upon the selection of appropriate goals, the 'personality' of the nurse acting as therapist and the relationship which she establishes with the patient. These intangible elements are often neglected in many textbooks which present a cook-book image, implying that the treatment method will work irrespective of how it is delivered. The role of the behaviour therapist is no different from that of any other therapist: she uses her personal qualities and professional skills and knowledge to influence the patient for the better. However, the way in which that interaction is structured may be different and may be characteristic of the behavioural approach. Nurse therapists, whether they are low-key presenters or highly skilled practitioners, provide the patient with information, aims, structure, help and feedback (see Figure 10.1). These 'provisions' are the practical outcome of the assessment, planning, intervention and evaluation stages described earlier.

Figure 10.1: The 'Giving' Components of Therapy

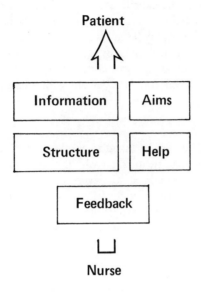

Information-giving

The nurse's first responsibility is to use assessment methods which are appropriate to the patient's problem. In many cases a standardised assessment system may be adapted slightly to suit the needs of the patient and his situation. In a minority of cases a special assessment may need to be devised. In either case the information collected should be a reliable and valid representation of the problem. The nurse uses this information to show the patient (or his significant others) whether the problem involves a behavioural excess or deficit, the extent of the problem and the factors which may be controlling it. The nurse also collects information about the patient's personal norms, his motivational state and his potential to control his own behaviour. The nurse's major aim in collecting and communicating this information, is to clear away any fuzziness surrounding the problem, some of which may have been put there by other well-intentioned people.

In information-giving the nurse tries to help the patient see his problem with a clear perspective. Where appropriate, he should be helped to see his difficulties as a function of his interaction with other people or events in his everyday life. Many patients are confused, frightened or embarrassed by the feelings or difficulties which they experience. Although she must never oversimplify the problem, the nurse tries to help the patient see his problem as it really is: devoid of mystery and mythology. Where the patient is unlikely to benefit from such a perspective, it may be to his advantage to offer this to his family or to those caring for him. By giving information the nurse may increase the patient's motivation to try to overcome the problem. This information will also provide him with a basis for evaluating his progress.

Aim-giving

Should the patient ever be asked to enrol for treatment without knowing what procedures, treatment goals, time-scale or personal effort is likely to be involved? In almost every case the answer would be an unequivocal 'No'. Where the patient cannot fully comprehend the nature of the treatment programme some significant other should speak on his behalf. In addition to describing the technical details of the treatment plan, the nurse should also give an estimate of the chances of success in achieving the treatment goals.

When the nurse is setting treatment goals she helps the patient, or his advocate, picture what might be a 'successful solution'. Some kind of 'cost–benefit analysis' must be carried out to ensure that any trauma involved in therapy is outweighed by the likely rewards of success. Figure 10.2 gives an example of a format which could be used to discuss the pros and cons of a possible treatment programme. In some situations (e.g. in hospitals) it may be helpful to record the decision to begin a treatment plan along the lines illustrated. In other settings (e.g. a community clinic) a simple note made by the nurse in the patient's progress notes may suffice. This discussion is used to clarify the exact nature of the aims of treatment: what is likely to be done, how and by whom. By giving explicit details of the aims of treatment, the nurse further reduces the mystique of therapy and encourages the participation of the patient or his significant others.

Structure-giving

The structure of the treatment programme influences the selection of treatment procedures. The structure is the medium for behaviour change. The structure may involve, at a very basic level, a task analysis of a single behaviour, e.g. of dressing or feeding behaviours. On a more comprehensive level a wide range of behaviours might be incorporated into a therapeutic *system*, such as a token economy or a social skills

Figure 10.2: Cost-benefit Analysis of Treatment Programme

DATE .6/8/81...

REF. BY
Dr. J.S. Jones

. . . .

CODE

030757

ANALYSIS OF BENEFIT – COST (A-B-C)

Analyse treatment proposal by comparison of BENEFITS likely to be gained, with COSTS required to be expended by 1, 2 & 3 below. The decision to implement, modify or reject the proposal should be taken by consensus opinion and recorded.

1: Subject BRIAN REDFORD............ Resident WILLOW WARD.

'Problem' MESSY EATER, REFUSES TO USE SPOON..........

Proposal INCREASE APPROPRIATE SPOON USE, DECREASE NOISY OUTBURSTS AT TABLE.

2: Significant 1. JANET, DICK & SANDRA..... Relationship CARE TEAM.

Others) 2. MRS. REDFORD........... Relationship MOTHER.....

3: Programme 1. SISTER DICKENS.......... Dept WILLOW WARD C/N

Supervisor(s) 2. MAY TODD............. Dept NURSE THERAPIST...

	BENEFITS	COSTS
SUBJECT	Could sit with others at table! could go into restaurants on town visits.	? Frustration Longer mealtimes Required to sit for longer
SIGNIFICANT OTHERS	(1+2) Job satisfaction (1) Reduction in supervision time at meals	(1+2) Time spent learning programme (1) Possible disruption of normal ward routines
PROGRAMME SUPERVISOR	(1+2) Job satisfaction (1) Demonstration of effectiveness of nursing team	(1) Time spent recording progress 2) Time spent teaching staff + 'on call' for problems in running Programme.

DECISION: BEGIN PROGRAMME AT EARLIEST OPPORTUNITY

APPROVED BY:
Dr. J.S. Jones

DATE 14/8/81.........

programme. The structure includes details of where, when and how the patient should perform the target behaviours. It also details staff management policies, where appropriate, and gives instructions about any adaptation to the patient's physical environment which may be necessary. This structure gives the patient a chance to practice, or rehearse, the target behaviours under optimum reinforcement conditions. These will be adapted gradually to approximate his natural environment or to help him progress to another stage of therapy. Once again, the explicit nature of the therapy structure gives the patient a clear idea of what will happen to him and what he will be expected to do in the treatment programme.

Help-giving

Help is never offered arbitrarily. Careful consideration should always be given to the kind of help *this* patient needs, as distinct from other patients with similar problems. The nurse should use herself as a therapeutic tool, providing clear and concise instructions, modelling the target behaviour and providing other kinds of assistance through verbal and non-verbal prompts, such as graduated guidance.

The kind of help required varies according to the nature of the patient's problem, the demands of the treatment method and the stage he has reached in therapy. As the programme progresses help will be faded, leaving the patient to operate more and more in a 'self-help' situation. In addition to this discrete interpersonal help, the nurse will also provide pieces of equipment − such as video or tape recorders − guidelines on the use of certain self-control procedures or instructions for homework assignments. She may also provide visual aids, such as signs and notices, or other items of equipment, such as special clothing or eating utensils. These 'aids' should be selected, or in some cases prepared specially for the patient, to ensure that the programme can continue when the nurse is not available to supervise or provide more direct forms of help: e.g. when the programme is delegated to some less expert 'therapist' such as a nursing aide or a parent.

Feedback-giving

How does the patient know that he is making progress? Is he moving towards, or away from, the targets which were set for him? To a great extent his awareness of progress or regression will be influenced by the kind of feedback he receives. On one level feedback can be defined as the immediate consequences of his behaviour. If he gives eye-contact, the nurse may reinforce this by smiling: 'non-verbal positive feedback'.

If she needs to be more explicit she may praise him, or issue some tangible form of reinforcement, such as a piece of food or a token. A patient like Sally, who has impaired memory function, may need to be prepared for the kind of feedback she can expect: 'When you do this Sally . . . this will happen.'

Feedback, on another level, involves informing the patient about how his behaviour has been 'received' by those around him. The nurse is helping the patient to know whether his behaviour is having the effect intended, whether or not he is 'on target'. These positive or negative comments about the patient's performance can be consolidated by providing him with graphs, charts, photographs or other recordings of 'progress'. Even with mentally handicapped children, simple charts recording their progress from one day to the next can be highly effective in promoting behaviour change.

The Human Relationship

Behaviour therapists do not, as often is commonly thought, dismiss the importance of the relationship with the patient. Indeed such a bond is crucial if the processes of information, aims, structure, help and feedback-giving are to achieve their ends. The basic doctrine of behaviourism underlines this point, emphasising the reciprocal relationship between the patient and his environment. If the patient is reinforced by the nurse, and vice versa, a good relationship will be in evidence and the success of therapy is more likely. If either party finds the other aversive, then the whole exercise will be abortive.

Emotional Distance. It is important for nurses to examine their feelings about the patient in order to establish an appropriate emotional distance. For some nurses this may mean establishing a 'one-sided relationship' with each and every patient. The nurse respects the patient and cares about his problems. However, she tries to avoid letting her personal values or feelings interfere with the course of therapy. If the patient is hostile or refuses to co-operate, our 'natural' reaction would be to express our displeasure or disappointment. In the one-sided relationship, the nurse makes a rule that she leave her personal views or opinions outside of the therapy situation. This approach, which involves refusing to become emotionally entangled with the patient, may be helpful when he is very disturbed or distressed. The nurse believes that her 'natural' reactions would only be a personal safety valve and may not help the patient. Instead, she aims for a more professional, and measured, reaction.

For other nurses, this approach may be unrealistic. Many nurses need to 'mother' handicapped children or to befriend psychiatric patients. The dangers of such close relationships are of course the hurt, unhappiness and frustration experienced when the patient fails to co-operate or does not meet the targets set. Many nurses argue that the costs are outweighed by the benefits likely to be accrued. No firm rulings can be given: each nurse must measure her own distance, perhaps adjusting this according to the patient concerned.

The Proficiency Approach. Throughout this book we have argued that a proficiency, rather than deficiency, model is the best way of looking at the patient. Instead of describing him as a collection of problems or weaknesses, why cannot we see him as someone with limited abilities which can be strengthened or extended? This positive outlook may be beneficial when working with severely disabled people and may be a natural antidote to the pessimism which many nurses feel when faced with the 'overkill' negative evaluations contained in many case reports. As we noted earlier, a major deficiency of the medical model is its almost wholly negative view of the patient. However, surely even the most profoundly disabled person can do something? Society uses the term 'vegetable' as a pejorative description of the most profoundly disabled. This is true irony, since vegetables are in a state of slow, yet constant 'personal growth': the human eye is simply unable to discern this. Nurses may be in a much better position to help the patient if they begin by analysing his positive attributes.

Confused Communications. Patients who are experiencing a severe crisis often find it difficult to communicate this to the nurse working with them. Are patients who fail to keep appointments at clinics rejecting help or experiencing a new difficulty? When a handicapped child is aggressive towards the nurse during a skills training session, is this a sign that he wants to get out of the situation? Is he being awkward, or is the level of proficiency demanded of him too high and causing him frustration? There is no easy way of identifying such intangible problems and there are certainly no easy solutions. However, the nurse must be alert to the possible reasons why patients fail to co-operate or appear to be withdrawing from the programme. They may be experiencing problems which can be resolved. They may be communicating something other than the obvious.

A Word About Caring. We could define 'caring' as doing unto others as we would have them do unto us. If that definition is correct, few of us would agree that all institutions, or nurses, are successful care-providers. Apart from 'doing' for the *patient*, caring also involves believing in him — believing that behind the mask of the patient label, or his condition, lies another unique human being, like ourselves. When we care for a patient, we embrace much more than the defective part which requires correction or modification: we embrace the whole individual. If we do not embrace the whole person we provide a very limited, technical service, in the same way as a garage mechanic changes a defective sparking plug. He is not 'servicing the car'; he is isolating and amending a single defective component, which may or may not be the root of the problem. Our 'service' to the patient is a total one, embracing all aspects of his behaviour, even those which we find difficult to accept or understand.

Therapeutic Attitudes

It would be inappropriate to discuss here the training of nurses in behaviour therapy. Different kinds of training programme are required, depending upon the level of expertise required. However, there may be some value in discussing some of the attitudinal problems which dog the practice of therapy, at all levels.

The Radical Behaviourist

As we have noted throughout this book, 'radical behaviourism' takes the view that only observable behaviour is important. What the patient thinks or feels about his problem is of little consequence. Some nurses follow this line believing that this is what *real* behaviourism is all about. More importantly, this model can be distinguished easily from other forms of 'psychotherapy', where the therapist discusses only experiences, analyses relationships and probably rolls around naked at some encounter group. Myths about the true nature of behaviourism and psychotherapy abound, and do not help to distinguish the practices. Few therapists practice 'radical' behaviour therapy, although many books are written as if this was the commonest approach.

Some nurses are attracted to behaviour therapy 'on the rebound' from a bad experience in another field of therapy. The cool logic or technology of behaviourism may appear more like common sense and may be more to their liking. However, if the nurse oversimplifies the patient's problems, or presents therapy in a mechanical fashion, the exercise is likely to be abortive. Patients often need 'support' as well as structure and 'encouragement' as well as reinforcement. At some stage in the programme the patient may want just to 'talk' to the nurse about what is happening to him. The nurse who sticks rigidly to a radical behaviourist format risks alienating the patient, who may be unhappy about returning for further sessions.

The Eclectic Therapist

The nurse working in behaviour therapy needs to be flexible. Some treatment methods which have a long pedigree are now overshadowed with doubt and may soon be replaced by new techniques. Change, within the approach itself, is a natural outcome of research into the viability of different ways of helping the patient. However, this does not mean that behaviour therapy has no central orientation or that 'anything goes'. The behaviour therapist tries to translate the tangled web, which is the patient's problem, into everyday terms which both nurse and patient can understand. Other therapies often weave even more intricate patterns as they analyse the patient's network of relationships and experiences. In àdvocating a 'broad-spectrum' approach to therapy, we are not saying that the nurse can 'change hats' whenever she feels like it. Any change in therapeutic style, or technique, must be part of the overall plan and should never be taken arbitrarily.

The Benefits of Therapy

Why do nurses want to practise behaviour therapy? Especially where they may know little about what it may involve, what are the nurse's motives for taking up this, as opposed to any other, therapy? Some nurses enrol for training, or volunteer to work in a behavioural ward, because they are unhappy with their current work. Behaviour therapy may look like a more exciting prospect. She can become a 'therapist' rather than remain just an 'ordinary nurse'. Although few nurses report that it is boring, the delivery of a carefully planned, and consistently applied, treatment programme is rarely all fun and excitement. Some procedures, such as relaxation training or shaping spoon use, are painstaking. When these are applied routinely, the demand for concentration and skill may increase rather than decrease The nurse must be always on the alert. Is the patient signalling difficulties? Which behaviours should I reinforce? Which should I punish? Do I need to revise the programme? Although successful therapy brings rewards to the nurse, especially when working with severely handicapped patients or those who are resistive to change, the work can be frustrating, repetitive and a lengthy process. Even where the nurse is given a formal 'therapist' title, the work may have little apparent glamour.

Nurses should ask themselves why they want to do behaviour therapy. Do they want to help the patient – and this seems like the best way? Do they want to extend their therapeutic skills? Or do they want to add some spice to what has now become a less than satisfying occupation? This last reason is one which often attracts people to work in any field of psychotherapy: the promise of being privy to intimate details about the patient, or having the satisfaction of dealing with patients which others cannot cope with. These kinds of thrills or satisfactions are natural; we are human first and nurses second. However, the nurse who will make a 'good therapist' may be less interested in the therapy for her own sake and may be more oriented towards the needs of the patient. Once again, the 'good caring nurse' and the good therapist are virtually indistinguishable.

The Last Resort

Some nurses come, or are sent, to behaviour therapy as a last resort. Senior staff often see behaviour therapy as a soft option, which does not demand the skills and intelligence necessary for group psychotherapy with alcoholics or running a therapeutic community for adolescents. Myths about the simplicity of behaviour therapy die hard and are reinforced each time someone establishes another token economy at the drop of a hat.

Acute admission wards or work with children are, traditionally, the glamour areas of psychiatric or mental handicap nursing. When nurses are sent to 'back wards' to work with chronic patients or the most severely mentally handicapped, they may interpret this as a punishment. If they are also obliged to participate in an alien activity like behaviour therapy or modification, this may only be adding insult to injury. Work with chronic patients or the more severely disabled needs the highest calibre of nurse, not the least expert or the apathetic. As we argued in Chapter 6, behaviour therapy should not be used to shore up deficiencies in the organisational structure of the hospital. The approach should be used to resolve the problems of the patient, not of the service which is meant to be caring for him. Where nurses are unwilling or unable to offer a therapeutic service, the imposition of a behavioural programme will change nothing. If these nurses are to be encouraged to adopt a new role, they must be given special support to help them change their attitudes towards certain patients, or to overcome their sense of worthlessness (whether real or imaginary) before embarking upon the task of helping others.

Summary

Nurses have a great potential to exert a positive influence on their patients. They are often in the best position to help the patient and may possess personal qualities which are lacking in other therapists. This potential is, however, rarely realised. Nurses often maintain the patient in a dependent state or may unwittingly foster his dependence. This situation may have its roots in the ill-defined and unsystematic nature of nurse–patient relationships. The confusion as to the meaning of the term 'care' has aggravated the problem and nurses have spent much time debating the care *versus* therapy issue, when both terms appear to be synonymous.

Although nurses began as the hoteliers of the asylum era and were then cultivated as doctor's assistants, nursing theorists claim that nursing is an independent activity, bringing its own brand of help to the patient. The aims of nursing have been defined in broad terms and the technology is now being studied within the concept of the process of nursing, a process which is complementary to the behavioural process. Its growth in popularity in the late 1970s augurs well for the increased acceptance of behaviour therapy in the 1980s.

Four specific role models have emerged within nurse behaviour therapy within the last decade. These represent: the nurse's role as the presenter of the programme; as its overall co-ordinator; the highly skilled, and independent, practitioner; and the nurse consultant, who acts as clinician, planner and researcher. Training programmes for presenters and co-ordinators are emerging, whereas schemes of training for the more specialist roles are now well-established.

The nurse's relationship with the patient involves providing him with information about his problem, discrete goals to aim for and a structure within which to achieve these therapeutic targets. Active help and evaluation of progress is given by delivery of specific behavioural techniques and giving of feedback. These technical skills are insufficient to ensure the success of the programme. The nurse must provide the patient with the care and understanding implicit in any therapy and must be prepared to recognise when she must develop her interpersonal skills or cultivate more appropriate attitudes towards the patient. To be a therapist, the nurse must show genuine concern for the patient. One way or another, she must get 'emotionally involved'.

Notes

1. Peck, D.F. 'An agent of behaviour change: the psychiatric nurse as therapist', *Nursing Times*, Occasional Paper (13 August 1973).

2. Marks, I.M., Hallam, R.S. and Philpott, R. 'Behavioural nurse therapists? The implications', *Nursing Times*, Occasional Paper (13 May 1976).

3. McPherson, F.M., Barker, P., Hunter, M. and Fraser, D. 'A course in behaviour modification', *Nursing Times* (20 July 1978).

4. Marks, I.M., Bird, J. and Lindley, P. 'Behavioural nurse therapists 1978 – developments and implications', *Behavioural Psychotherapy*, vol. 6 (1978), pp. 25-36.

5. Ginsberg, G. and Marks, I.M. 'Costs and benefits of behavioural psychotherapy: a pilot study of neurotics treated by nurse-therapists', *Psychological Medicine*, vol. 7 (1977), pp. 320-1.

6. Walsh, P.A. ' "Mental Illness", "mental handicap" and the nursing service establishment – an alternative approach', *Journal of Advanced Nursing*, vol. 1 (1976), pp. 283-92.

7. Quoted on p. 327 of Bird, J., Marks, I.M. and Lindley, P. 'Nurse therapists in psychiatry: developments, controversies and implications', *British Journal of Psychiatry*, vol. 135 (1979), pp. 321-9.

8. This view was expressed by LeBow, M.D. 'Applications of behaviour modification in nursing practice', In: M. Hersen, R.M. Eisler and P. Miller (eds), *Progress in Behaviour Modification, Vol. 2*.(New York, Academic Press, 1976).

9. Ayllon, T. and Michael, J. 'The psychiatric nurse as a behavioural engineer', *Journal of the Experimental Analysis of Behaviour*, vol. 2 (1959), pp. 323-34.

10. Gelfand, D., Gelfand, S. and Dobson, W.R. 'Unprogrammed reinforcement of patients' behaviour in a mental hospital', *Behaviour Research and Therapy*, vol. 5 (1967), pp. 201-7.

11. Ibid., p. 205.

12. Cormack, D. and Fraser, D. 'The nurse's role in psychiatric institutions', *Nursing Times*, Occasional Paper (25 December 1975).

13. Simpson, R. 'Psychiatric nursing – what now?' *Nursing Times* (5 June 1980).

14. Scottish National Nursing & Midwifery Consultative Committee, 'A new concept of nursing', *Nursing Times*, Occasional Paper (8, 15 & 22 April 1976).

15. Davis, B. 'Why do we need the nursing process? 3. For professional reasons', *Nursing Times* (30 November 1978).

16. Ashworth, P., Castledine, G. and McFarlane, J.K. 'Rediscovering the patient. The process in practice', *Nursing Times Supplement* (30 November 1978).

17. Crow, J. *The Nursing Process* (London, Macmillan Journals, 1977).

18. Barker, P. Letters, *Nursing Times* (25 October 1979).

19. LeBow, In: *Progress in Behaviour Modification*, pp. 137-77.

20. Horne, D.J., de L., McTiernan, G. and Strauss, N.H.M. 'A case of severe obsessive -compulsive behaviour treated by nurse therapists in an in-patient unit', *Behavioural Psychotherapy*, vol. 9 (1981), pp. 46-54.

21. McPherson, F.M., Cockram, L.K., Grimes, J., Fraser, D. and Presly, A.S. 'The restoration of one aspect of communication in chronic psychiatric patients', *Health Bulletin* (September 1979).

22. Hall, J.N. and Rosenthal, G. 'Operant treatment of the long-term patient', *Nursing Times* (6 September 1973), pp. 143-8.

23. Barker, P. 'Handicaps in perspective', *Nursing Mirror* (27 November 1975).

24. Kiernan, C.C. and Riddick, B. 'A draft programme for training in operant techniques' (University of London, Institute of Education, 1973).

25. Orwin, A. 'Psychiatric nurses as behavioural therapists', *Nursing Times*, vol. 72 (1976), pp. 461-4.

26. Stoffelmayer, B.E., Lindsay, W. and Taylor, V. 'Maintenance of staff behaviour', *Behaviour Research and Therapy*, vol. 17 (1979), pp. 271-3.

27. Duberly, J. 'The clinical nurse specialist', *Nursing Times* (18 November 1976).

28. Schmidt, M.P.W. and Duncan, B.A.B. 'Modifying eating behaviour in anorexia nervosa', *Am. Journal of Nursing*, vol. 74 (1974), pp. 1646-8.

29. Brookes, D.J. and Brown, C.A. 'A behavioural approach to rehabilitation', *Nursing Times* (26 February 1981).

30. Barker, P. 'Behaviour therapy in psychiatric and mental handicap nursing', *Journal of Advanced Nursing*, vol. 5 (1980), pp. 55-69.

31. Marks, Bird and Lindley, *Behavioural Psychotherapy*, vol. 6, pp. 25-36.

11 AN EPILOGUE

All sciences are vain and full of errors that are
not born of experience, mother of all certainty,
and that are not tested by experience.
— Leonardo da Vinci

A Personal Viewpoint

In this book I have tried to paint a fair picture of contemporary behaviour therapy. I have described an approach which is practised by a
small, yet growing, band of nurses. I have included, also, reference to
therapeutic methods or attitudes which are of relevance to nursing
practice. In this chapter I should like to address some of the loose ends
which I have tried to tie up at various points in the book. These issues
— some ethical, some philosophical and some the subject of academic
debate — are likely to remain unfinished business for some time to
come. Although my picture of behaviour therapy is a fair one, it is
tainted with my own biases. I am aware of three prejudices, in particular, which, given the existing evidence or climate of opinion, may make
me appear irrational or unduly romantic.

First, I am aware that I have given the social learning theoretical
model, and certain 'relationship' variables, more emphasis than some of
my colleagues would have expected. My expressions of doubt in the
'established conditioning models', coupled with the exclusion or
underrating of certain treatment methods, may suggest to some that I
have 'gone soft'. Although I have acknowledged that firm evidence for
some of the approaches which I have advocated is only emerging, the
view to which I subscribe is well established. I have merely extended
the argument for a broader theoretical model and more 'holistic' care
and treatment, to include *all* patient groups in the mental field. I
believe that an 'inclusive' (as opposed to 'reductionist') view of our
patients is an essential ingredient of any care plan. Although frequently
neglected or misrepresented, the role of mediational processes and
attention to 'relationship' factors must be taken seriously by all nurses
wishing to present comprehensive care to any patient population.

Secondly, I have indulged my passion for supporting the underdog.
I have expressed the hope that a more humanistic care and treatment
model will soon be available to all severely mentally handicapped or
chronic psychiatric patients. Two of the patient 'stereotypes' who

appeared in the text were offered just such a treatment plan: I only wish that more nurses were willing to translate therapeutic possibilities into everyday clinical reality. I argued, also, that such patients must be seen as being, at least, as complex as ourselves. I believe that this plain truth is evidenced, in one respect, by our consistent failure to help them on a scale commensurate with their problems. Instead of implying their inferior status on the human scale, we should confront our anxieties and weaknesses, in an attempt to repair the gulf we have created.

Thirdly, I have stretched my definition of 'behaviour' very wide indeed, accommodating almost every conceivable human action under that umbrella title. Although this may not conform to some people's view of behaviourism, this is the subject matter which we are all faced with, day in and day out. I confess that my picture of behaviour therapy is painted with a broad brush, often in sweeping strokes, in an impressionistic style. The image on the canvas remains, none the less, that of behaviour therapy as it is commonly practised.

I believe that my prejudices for acknowledgement of the need for a broader-based therapy are becoming well-established. In the same vein I expect all nurses, sooner or later, to study behaviour in its widest sense: encompassing all aspects of the human condition. On a less positive note I fear that my craving for fair play for the more severely disabled patient may never be satisfied; for some the act of helping must be supplemented with all the pompous trappings of public charity.

What is Behaviour Therapy?

Lost Among the Titles

The practice of behaviour therapy has grown rapidly in the past decade. This often leads to confusion, for practitioner and onlooker alike. What, exactly, is behaviour therapy? What began as the application of modern stimulus-response learning theory is now practised by a range of disciplines, incorporating inputs from all corners of behavioural science. New titles also abound: community behaviour therapy, cognitive behaviour therapy, holistic behaviour therapy, behavioural medicine, self-directive behaviour therapy, multimodal behaviour therapy, are only a few of the labels which have surfaced of late.[1] In the best tradition of political rivalry, if not religious fervour, each claims to be the spearhead of *the* new behaviour therapy.

Nurses should not be too concerned with labels, or academic arguments as to the rightful heir to the behavioural throne. Behaviour therapy cannot be explained totally by any one theoretical model. Given the range of problems and treatment settings, it is only natural, also, that a string of variations on the basic theme should develop. The success of behaviour therapy depends, also, on a number of factors which have little, if anything, to do with learning theory. Anyone who aims only to 'condition' or 'decondition' behaviour is likely to be hugely unsucccessful. The recognition that there is more to behaviour therapy than conditioning is reflected in both research and clinical literature. The therapist's *relationship* with the patient has been studied closely.[2] Others have acknowledged that the patient's *expectations* may play a large part in influencing the outcome of treatment.[3] On the clinical front, therapists have tried to add to their 'tool kit' by adapting techniques from other fields. Arnold Lazarus is most famous in this respect, through his introduction of techniques and values from humanistic psychology.[4]

The decision to widen the range of available skills, or to cultivate our awareness of the importance of the therapeutic relationship, was not taken lightly. It has long been recognised that the effective therapist must be able to *present* the solution: knowing the answer is not enough. As behaviour therapy forges its new image in the 1980s, it is deeper and more intricate than its narrowly defined ancestor which emerged on to the clinical scene twenty-five years ago. Some nurses may be disappointed that this simplicity has been rejected, especially those who were attracted by the apparently easy answers the early model had on offer. Although the contemporary model is more intricate, this does not mean that it is becoming obscure. To pretend that behaviour is a simple affair is to practise self-deception. An appreciation of the many determinants of behaviour — genetic, biological, environmental and cognitive — should help us to see our patients, and ourselves, in a clearer light.

Justified Criticisms

The public birth of behaviourism was an aggressive affair, with J.B. Watson's outrageous views upon what was, or was not, suitable subject matter for the study of human behaviour. This aggressive posture was revived many years later by the radical behaviourists, led by B.F. Skinner, who is accredited with being the founding father of behaviour therapy and modification. Skinner's writings have earned him both plaudits and hostile criticism from the humanitarian lobby. It is often difficult for the uninitiated to establish what, exactly,

Skinner stands for, or what the fuss has been all about. Perhaps he is most infamous for his views that behaviourism has no ethical basis and that it is *the* scientific study of human behaviour. His philosophical views have been criticised as dangerous nonsense, likely to provide fodder for a totalitarian state,[5] and his 'scientific' model has been described as naive and simplistic. These criticisms are based on Skinner's irritating habit of discussing *human* behaviour, in the light of his experiments with *animals*. As his critics have pointed out, people and animals differ to the extent that man uses language to mediate his actions. Consequently, Skinner's plans for the social control and development of behaviour[6] along operant conditioning lines have all the hallmarks of a grandiose flight of fancy.

These criticisms have more than academic relevance. Some behaviour therapists have translated operant principles directly into treatment policies, especially in institutions. This naive use of experimental learning theory has often led to disastrous clinical results. Although Skinner is portrayed as the father of behaviour therapy and is an experimental psychologist of immense stature, one must reserve judgement as to the relevance of his views to behaviour therapy, as it is currently practised. The many criticisms which have been brought to bear, over the last two decades, would appear to suggest that many practitioners have listened carefully to the criticisms made and taken action to repair the breach where appropriate.

Keeping Alive the Myth

In spite of widespread exposure therapy is still greatly misunderstood. The popular myth represents it as a narrow and restrictive practice. Although the range of titles and influences of the past decade contrafict this viewpoint, many writers cling to its 'conditioning' image, emphasising the role of manipulative rewards or aversion, with Skinner acting as godfather to the unsavoury crew of change-agents. In other fields of nursing this would be akin to describing medicine as 'giving a patient a tablet to make him feel better' or surgery as 'dissecting the patient' — not incorrect, but misleading in its crass oversimplification.

Even at the time of writing nursing authors continue to perpetuate this myth, stirring up at the same time the adolescent — and outmoded — rivalry between psychotherapy and behaviourism. In one such article[7] a successful, but restrictive, operant treatment of encopretic children was used to illustrate the behavioural approach. Taking exception to some of the attitudes expressed in the report by a psychologist, the author concludes that most nurses might take the view that 'even if it works, I don't want to know'. She then issues an emotional appeal to nurses to fulfil their role *best*, and by implication to reject behaviour therapy, '. . . by retaining the traditional nursing attitude: an accepting, caring and non-judgemental one'. Attempts such as this to contrast the humanitarian stance of nursing with the cold and clinical approach of behaviourism, are typical of attempts to discredit behaviour therapy unfairly. The projection of the nurse as 'caring, accepting and non-judgemental', stems back to the nursing work of Sisters of Charity in the Middle Ages. Although such an attitude may be fitting for the religious life, there is little evidence that it represents the *best* role for the nurse. The results of Gelfand's study (15 years ago!) testify to the hazards of such an approach and illustrate the dangerous naivety inherent in treating all patients as though they were alike. Examples, such as the one cited, are often well-packaged media exercises, which communicate with an audience far larger than that reached by 'scientific' publications. Sadly, such a diet of half-truths serves only to perpetuate the myth and may deter many nurses from examining the 'facts' at first hand.

Who Cares Anyway?

Another common myth is the portrayal of the behaviour therapist as an emotionless technician, illustrated by the fatuous distinction between those 'who care' and those 'who change', as though they were mutually exclusive. The behaviour therapist may, however, be more *discriminating* in her dealings with the patient.

Mahoney[8] distinguishes between *sincere* and *manipulative* relationships with the patient. The 'caring' nurse might give praise when it is not due, 'to avoid hurting his feelings', or might encourage the patient to underestimate the extent of a problem 'to ease his distress'. Mahoney is sceptical of the ethics of such action, as he might be of the nurse who rejects an effective treatment method out of hand. He warns that this may lead the patient into even more painful discoveries in the future, when he discovers the real extent of his abilities or the enormity of his problems. Encouragement is a central issue in behaviour therapy, whether it is called reinforcement or not. Encouragement should, however, be realistic and delivered with sincerity. Gelfand showed us the danger of offering support indiscriminately.

Why Practise Behaviour Therapy?

The Clinical Model

The practice of behaviour therapy, as described in this book, may be frustrating for some, since I have avoided offering standard solutions for common problems. Many nurses look to behaviour therapy for a solution to incontinence or aggression, expecting to be given a behavioural aspirin which they can then issue to a whole range of patients. Reality, like the patient himself, is more complicated. A problem which is common to several patients may have different roots or maintaining factors. Unless these are revealed then appropriate treatment cannot be given. This underlines the need for adequate and skillful assessment, a point which has been stressed *ad nauseam* throughout the text.

If the patient suffers, for example, from insomnia, a number of factors could be maintaining 'staying awake'. The patient's biological clock may be upset and he might benefit from a more regular rising and retiral routine. He may also be engaging in behaviour which competes with falling asleep, e.g. reading or smoking in bed, or dozing in an armchair in the evening. If this is the case some kind of stimulus control programme may be indicated. The patient may need specific cues to prepare him for sleep, such as a set retiral routine, or may be gaining reinforcement from family or friends for his insomnia. On a different level he may be experiencing tension which inhibits sleep. An exercise routine earlier in the day, or a relaxation session before retiring, may help overcome this problem. Finally, his problem may be on a 'mental' level; the patient may be preoccupied with worries or may be worrying about his insomnia. Perhaps he has unhelpful beliefs, such as 'I need a good eight hours sleep every night'. These beliefs or his other worries will need to be tackled directly to solve the insomnia.

A problem may exist on any one of a number of levels, from the biological to the cognitive. Each requires a different solution. However, before we can solve it, we must know what the problem is: again, we are back to the need for careful assessment. Although behaviour therapy is often accused of oversimplifying people, there is a danger that the unsophisticated therapist may try to take in too much of the person. Indeed, other approaches which suggest that all problems of living are rooted in sexual hang-ups, or the result of unresolved interpersonal problems, may be more guilty of oversimplifying man.

I have argued that the way of looking at human problems of living, illustrated in the insomnia example above, is of great relevance to nurses working in the psychiatric or mental handicap fields. The open-ended nature of the approach allows the nurse to accommodate methods and values from other branches of the 'helping arts'. In order to practise behaviour therapy, a nurse need not blind herself to the potential value of other approaches. Indeed, the fewer people wearing blinkers in the field, the better the standard of care and treatment.

Considering the Evidence

Some authors have argued that behaviour therapy is unsuitable for the majority of 'neurotic disorders'.[9] By implication, this means that it is unsuitable for those experiencing more severe problems of living. Although research has shown that behaviour therapy is the *treatment of choice* for phobic, obsessive-compulsive, social skill problems, sexual dysfunction and enuresis, other writers have argued that a variety of behavioural approaches hold great promise for widespread problems (such as cognitive therapy and depression) and the approach has a great deal to offer the mental field as a whole.[10] This cautious optimism is reinforced by the awareness that alternative approaches have little to offer these patients.

Although behaviour therapy can be hugely successful when applied *alone*, it has a valuable role to play as an adjunct therapy. Marital problems and interpersonal problems can be helped when behaviour therapy is offered in conjunction with other systems of support. The same is true of some patients suffering from the effects of alcohol abuse. Severe cases of generalised anxiety can also be treated where the behavioural programme is synchronised with a carefully controlled course of medication. The patient who is so disturbed or handicapped that he needs hospitalisation, has few therapeutic facilities open to him. Drugs, custodial care and a short period of occupational therapy, are often the only 'treatments' available; yet none of these is renowned for its ability to restore or instil the social or interpersonal skills which the patient needs. In this situation behavioural approaches have a great role to play as an adjunct therapy, but are, as yet, a largely untapped resource.

A Viable Technology

One of the key attractions of behaviour therapy must be its techno-logical sophistication. Although only at a primitive stage of development, a technology for resolving a number of problems of living is growing. Hopefully, this technology will soon progress from a wholly 'curative' basis, to accommodate some 'preventative' work. In addition to dealing with problems as they arise, the approach could be used to help people ward off crises (e.g. helping people cope with stress) or to aid the design of special training programmes for the severely disabled. Although the success of current efforts is encouraging, it often looks like 'too little — too late'.

In view of the relative lack of effective therapeutic skills shown by nurses in the field, the behavioural approach looks like a godsend. I have tried to illustrate the breadth of assessment and treatment methods available and have shown how these can be used by nurses with even limited skills or experience. Although a sophisticated person is needed to plan and direct programmes, or to present them in certain situations, the basic technology is within the grasp of most nurses. Disappointingly, many nurses continue to look this particular gift horse in the mouth.

Where is Behaviour Therapy Going?

The Cognitive Bogey

The gradual increase of interest in the role of mediational processes was stimulated by Bandura, but has been reinforced by the development of specific cognitive techniques, especially by Meichenbaum and Beck. Given that some therapists may have believed stoically that 'thinking' was beyond their terms of reference, it is not surprising that the increased use of cognitive methods has generated something of an identity crisis. Some writers[11] have argued that behaviour therapists have always used cognitive methods, in conjunction with overt behavioural practices. Although the therapist may talk to the patient, and answer any questions about his problems, this is in no way similar to the methods of self-instruction or cognitive restructuring. Cognitions have always played some part in certain practices, such as desensitisation or thought-stopping. Their role, however, was very much a background affair. Consequently, the adoption of these new techniques and the interest in all things cognitive signifies a new, and stimulating, development.

Much of the reaction to cognitive methods stems back to behaviourism's early rejection of 'inferred variables' and the whole tradition of 'mentalism' (see Chapter 2). However, the rejection of inferences about cognitive processes can hardly by substantiated on scientific grounds. Established sciences, like physics, have used highly extravagant inferences, in order to construct their theoretical models, e.g. quantum theory. Since the early behaviourists were keen to establish themselves on the same footing as the physicists, this makes the unease of present-day radical behaviourists, over mediational processes, seem a little odd.

The exact role of cognition as a determinant of behaviour seems to be unclear. What is apparent is that people do study their own behaviour in relation to the world around them, do remember what has happened to them in the past and do anticipate what may happen in the future. We have nothing to gain, and much to lose, by ignoring this fact. As Bandura has argued,[12] behaviour is not shaped and regulated *solely* by external influences. Environmental factors interlock with a person's behaviour, his thinking and other 'individual differences', to determine his actions. The search for a single factor to explain why we behave the way we do, is like a search for the psychological Grail. However, to acknowledge that people can exert *some* influence over their own behaviour, does not raise the spectre of autonomous man. Instead it will lead to research which will deepen our understanding of how the environment and the person interact to determine human behaviour.[13]

Fostering the Personal Scientist

I have suggested that the role of the nurse is an educational one. She helps the patient learn more about his 'condition' and how to cope with the events which upset, frustrate or defeat him. This educational model is applicable to the incontinent child, as much as it is to the anxious adult. The 'therapist' is not so much a healer, as a provider of the structure whch the patient needs to resolve his difficulties. Mahoney has elaborated upon this idea in his concept of the *personal scientist*.[14] He argues that the most 'humane' approach in goal-setting is to offer the patient a broad range of coping skills, which he can use to resolve his own difficulties. The approach involves the following seven stages:

(1) The patient is encouraged to look upon therapy as a problem-solving exercise. He is encouraged to view his problems as the result of a combination of events, some coming from his environment and some from 'within' himself. He is encouraged to assume responsibility for correcting his 'problem', with the therapist acting as a technical consultant, rather than healer. In this first phase, all attention is focused upon the patient's expectations.

(2) The patient is trained to define his complaint more clearly. The categories of behavioural excess and deficit are used, in addition to qualitative measures, e.g. 'unsatisfactory performance' or 'lack of incentive'.

(3) The patient is shown how to examine his problem in more detail, through systematic record-keeping. He records his behaviour,

its antecedents and consequences, and also his self-statements and personal standards.

(4) Once the problem has been analysed possible solutions are considered. Here, the therapist's technical role comes to the fore. In the main, *general*, coping skills — such as relaxation, covert modelling or coping self-instructions — are offered, rather than specific treatments, like desensitisation.

(5) In this phase the patient tests out a solution, in the form of an 'experiment'. A period of two weeks, at least, is taken to evaluate the effect of the exercise.

(6) Patient and therapist then evaluate progress. If the patient views this positively, then the approach is refined further. If he is dissatisfied, then the approach is modified in an attempt to come up with another solution.

(7) In the final phase the patient is gradually 'weaned off' the therapist. Mahoney recognises that even where efforts are made to prevent this, some dependence may develop.

Mahoney aknowledges that this approach is best suited to the less severely disturbed adult, who is still in the community. He argues, however, that the model can be adapted to suit children, adolescents and a range of institutionalised people. In particular, he notes that the ability to acquire problem-solving skills is *not* correlated strongly with intelligence. My own work, and that of many of my students, would seem to confirm this.

The idea of a 'personal scientist' is not fitting for all patients. Many might respond, however, to the challenge to do some 'detective work' on their problem. Where the patient is not already hospitalised, the approach goes a long way to maintaining his independence and self-respect. Where more chronic patients are involved, such an approach might restore a lot of dignity. Of course, this therapeutic style demands more effort and ingenuity. The desensitisation illustration in Chapter 8 — where the child was encouraged to imagine that he was meeting Superman — is typical of the creative programming necessary in work with children. The severely mentally handicapped, or the long-term psychiatric patient, might be thankful for a programme which aims to help him *and* to respect his individuality.

Who Are We and What Are We Doing Here?

Man the Clever Ape

One of the intriguing events of 1981 was the rebirth of anti-Darwinism in the United States. Plaintiffs appeared in several courts, arguing that the teaching of Darwin's evolutionary theory was usurping the religious freedom of their children. The rebirth of this debate, long since dead, led me to consider the nature of man, and our relationship with the animal kingdom.

References to animal experiments, and theories of human behaviour based upon animal studies, are peppered throughout this book. In this chapter I noted that our use of language is often used to distinguish man from other animals. We also suggest that animals have no higher consciousness: we think about our life and perhaps our death; we experience our own experience; we are *self*-conscious. We have long assumed that all animals lack this facility. The idea was born, so to speak, in the Book of Genesis, when Adam became *aware* of his own nakedness only after eating the apple of the tree of knowledge. However, recent work with chimpanzees seems to suggest that some of our assumptions about the difference between man and apes (at least) may be unfounded.[15] At the State University of New York, chimpanzees were confined in a cage with a full-length mirror. After the chimpanzee had become used to its image, it was put to sleep and an odourless dye was painted on parts of its body. The chimpanzee's reactions were then observed. After treating the 'new' image in the mirror as though it were a stranger, the chimp lost interest. However, it returned later and began to *study* its reflection in the mirror, grooming its eyes and mouth and picking its teeth, while studying the reflection. The studies showed not only that some apes could use complex language, such as sign-systems, but also that they appeared to be *self*-conscious.

This finding may surprise some people and not others. True to their fashion, some humans will refuse to accept the evidence, whereas others will ask 'What do we gain by knowing that?' I believe that such findings are important not because they tell us that some apes are more complex than we once believed, but because they help dispel a myth which prevents us understanding the animal world fully and which may have distorted our view of ourselves. The analogy with the study of human behaviour should be obvious. For generations we invented a wealth of fictions to account for various patterns of behaviour. When scientists attempt to explain some aspects of behaviour, or to dispel some of the age-old myths, we rarely express appreciation.

Zoologists, such as Desmond Morris, have done us a great service by studying man as though he were just another animal. On a wider scale, ethologists like Konrad Lorenz[16] have drawn comparisons between human behaviour and that of much lower-order species and have suggested that our very 'humanity' may prove to be our undoing.

The Art of Therapy

If we are in any doubt as to what we are, we should be in no doubt as to what we are doing here, at least in the professional sense. Throughout this book I have discussed behaviour therapy as a specialised form of 'helping'. The approach has its own distinctive style, but can, where required, blend with other helping techniques and agencies. Such help can be offered on a number of levels, from the technical to the sophisticated. All helpers are united by their concern for the patient, shown through their care and compassion. Helping is an expression of humanitarian concern. I hope I have not overstated my case for the recognition of behaviour therapy as a power for 'good' in the nursing field. However, I am aware that many people see behaviourism and humanism as strange bedfellows, if not wholly incompatible.

Skinner proposed the view that behavioural technology was not concerned with ethics and this has taken a lot of living down. Not only must the technology of behaviourism be scrutinised with care, but — more importantly — the values which lie behind the whole idea of behaviour change and control must be examined. Anyone who wishes to change behaviour, whether she is a behaviourist or not, must question her reasons and assumptions, for wanting — or daring — to do so.

The practice of behaviour therapy is linked strongly with the scientific tradition. However, I would suggest that for the nurse, at least, the idea of practising therapy *in the name of science* may be overambitious. The clinic, ward or shopping precinct differ greatly from the learning laboratory. Similarly, the control which the nurse exercises in these settings is often as much magical, as it is scientific. Nursing is largely an 'artistic' affair, although the same could be said of some aspects of behaviour therapy. The help a nurse offers in a behavioural programme is skillful and measured, since it is based upon the principles and technology which have been given to her. However, the way in which the help is *presented* is a complex affair, relying more on human judgement than scientific know-how. Were behaviour therapy wholly scientific, we could programme a computer to treat the patient or could guarantee our results each and every time. To say that therapy is not scientific, is not the overt criticism which it sounds. Although science and 'art' are now seen as poles apart, this was not always the case, as the record of men like Da Vinci shows. There is no reason why the human values and skills of helping, cannot co-exist with the science of human behaviour.

The drive towards the development of a 'behavioural humanism' should prove attractive to most nurses. In such an activity they will gain greater understanding of the aetiology of behaviour and will find a technology which can be manipulated and applied with ease and a set of values which will allow them to continue practising the art of nursing. It was once thought that a man could not believe in God and be a scientist. I hope that nurses do not make the same error by assuming that they cannot believe in man and be behaviourists.

Notes

1. From: Franks, C.M. '2081: will we be many or one – or none?' *Behavioural Psychotherapy*, vol. 9 (1981), pp. 287–90.

2. Goldfried, M.R. and Davidson, G.C. *Clinical Behaviour Therapy* (New York, Holt, Rinehart & Winston, 1976).

3. Kazdin, A.E. and Wilcoxen, L.A. 'Systematic desensitisation and non-specific treatment effects: a methodological evaluation', *Psychological Bulletin*, vol. 83 (1976), pp. 729–58.

4. Lazarus, A.A. 'Multimodal behaviour therapy: treating the basic "ID" ', *Journal of Nervous and Mental Disease*, vol. 156 (1973), pp. 404–11.

5. Chomsky, N. 'The case against B.F. Skinner', *The New York Review* (30 December 1971).

6. Skinner, B.F. *Beyond Freedom and Dignity* (Harmondsworth, Penguin, 1973).

7. Ross, T. 'Thought control', *Nursing Mirror* (23 April 1981).

8. Mahoney, M.J. *Cognition and Behaviour Modification* (Cambridge, Mass., Ballinger, 1974), p. 281.

9. Marks, I.M. 'Behavioural concepts and treatments of neuroses', *Behavioural Psychotherapy*, vol. 9 (1981), pp. 137–54.

10. Wilson, G.T. 'Behavioural concepts and treatments of neuroses: comments on Marks', *Behavioural Psychotherapy*, vol. 9 (1981), pp. 155–66.

11. Wolpe, J. 'Cognition and causation in human behaviour and its therapy', *American Psychologist*, vol. 35 (1978), pp. 437–46.

12. Bandura, A. 'In search of pure unidirectional determinants', *Behaviour Therapy*, vol. 12, no. 1 (1981), pp. 30–40.

13. Ibid., p. 38.

14. Mahoney, *Cognition and Behaviour Modification*, pp. 267–86.

15. Laidler, K. *The Talking Ape* (London, Collins, 1980).

16. Lorenz, K. *Civilized Man's Eight Deadly Sins* (London, Methuen, 1974).

APPENDIX 1

B.I.A.S.

BEHAVIOURAL INTERVIEW AND ANALYSIS SCHEDULE.

REF. CODE 140748   PRIORITY B   ACTION DATE 17/11/80

NAME NORA SMITH   AGE 32   D.O.B. 14/7/48

HOME ADDRESS 4, ERICT PLACE

     LARAWAY   TEL. 27219

WARD ____ DATE OF ADMISSION ____ Nº PREV. ADMISS. ____

MARITAL STATUS Seperated DEPENDENTS NONE

N.O.K. MRS. B. ADAMSON   RELATION MOTHER

ADDRESS 27, ANDERSON GARDENS

     STONFORTH   TEL. 44613

REFERRED BY DR. K. SOMMERS (G.P.)   DATE 24/10/80

ASSESSED BY JEAN KIRKWALL (Community)   DATE 19/11/80

CO-ORDINATOR (ABOVE)

© P. Barker 1979

–1–

<u>Referred Problem</u>   Panic attacks in shops. Frightened to leave house at times. Conflicts with Mother who she is currently staying with.

Diagnosis: Anxiety neurosis   agoraphobia

Handicaps – Motor: _____   Visual: Wears spectacles

Auditory: _____   Other: _____

Current Medical Treatment: 10 mg Nitrazepam   Nocte
                           5 mg Diazepam   T. I. D.

Personal History

Occupation: Personal Secretary at Jennings Holdings (Off sick for last 4 months.)

Social Background: Only child, married to accountant (Dick) seperated. living with Mother (Mrs Adamson)

Habits — Eating: Appetite normal   Sleeping: Difficulty getting off to sleep. Dreams about mother & shopping.

Social: Never goes out - Cause of friction with husband specially related to his work.   Sexual: Relations with husband were O.K. (now of course suspended)

Assets: Organised, Punctual, loyal & hard-working.

Deficits: Weak always been a 'softy'

Comments: Very tense during interview little sustained eye-contact. Clutching handbag throughout. Would not take her coat off. Tearful at any mention of her Mother. (Father deceased)

<u>Initial Problem Evaluation:</u>
Mrs. Smith feels guilty about being off work for so long. She believes that her employers may sack her. She spends a lot of time worrying about the future and dreading 'having to go out' when she is out of the house she thinks that she will collapse. Sometimes this passes off but only recedes when she gets back home again. Her Mother advises her constantly to pull herself together.

- 2 -

Problem History

A) Description: (1) PANIC ATTACKS. When out she is tense all the time. In certain shops and in the shopping complex she panics and must get out especially where there are a lot of people. She feels the same way when she has to speak to people

Previous Therapy: Valium   Date Current

Outcome: Little relief. Increased dosage & usage.

B) Frequency Every time she goes out! - has not been out socially for over a year.

Intensity   Getting worse over the last year.

Duration   Attacks last only a few minutes 'I just run home!'

C) Locations Large shops, work, canteen

Situations Eating in public Having to talk to Mr. Jacob's clients.

Persons Where there are a lot of people. My mother. Mr. Jacobs (Boss) Some shop assistants.

Materials Need to hold something smokes a lot to calm nerves Often drinks Vodka

D) Norms

Personal

Has always been 'nervy' Had few friends at school. This fear of going into crowds began after Dad died. Very close to him. Couldn't go to funeral.

Cultural

Fear of being sacked if she does not go back soon. Needs to arrange small functions as part of job

Social

Appreciate that a lot of people don't like crowds but can tolerate them. Neighbours say that she needs treatment Family think she doesn't help herself

– 3 –

Problem Analysis

Antecedents

Physical At the office, in shops, in a company (party)

Social People speaking all at once. Complaining to me or asking me to do a lot of things at once (Mr. Jacobs)

Behavioural Just stand listening   look for a way out.

Cognitive I must get out of here! I can't stand this! I don't know what to do!

Physiological Heart thumping, feel my legs like jelly. Can't think straight.

Consequences

Physical In toilet, out into street, into house.

Social Mother gives me tea to calm me down. Jacobs sends me to the rest room sometimes

Behavioural Lie down Have a cigarette. Sometimes take a drink at home after a row with Mum.

Cognitive I'm never going to get over this. I'm a mess. I am weak

Physiological   Quite calm

PROBLEM DEFINITION 'Avoidance of social situations' has developed over the last two years. Significant situations are work, shops and any meeting with strangers. When people 'put pressure' on her she freezes, doesn't know how to handle the situation and feels she must escape. Feels better as soon as she has escaped. Feigns sickness to avoid 'contacts' at work or hides in toilet. Gets a lot of support from understanding boss and mother after these attacks.
     Suffers recrimination soon afterwards.

– 4 –

Motivational Analysis (A)

Consumables: (Likes)	(Dislikes)
Cigarettes, Vodka, Cakes, Chocolates	Mum's cooking

| Tangibles : | |
| Clothes, records (classical) books pot plants. | Radio + T.V. (noisy rubbish) |

People :

    Jean Davidson (Old school friend)   Mother (sometimes. I know
    Dick   (Husband)   she tries to help but . . . . .)
    Dad (Deceased)   Mrs Brown (admin typist)
    Barbara (from the office)

Places :

    The garden   shops (Superstores)
    bedroom (quiet)   crowded streets
    park (sometimes)

Activities: Reading, listening to   Repetetive things (files etc)
records, gardening, cookery.

PREFERENCE RANKING

1) Listening to music (Greig, McCunn)	1) Crowds
2) Smoking	2) Shops
3) Cooking for friends	3) Repetition
4) Reading (good novels non fiction)	

– 5 –

Motivational Analysis   (B)

Independence

I need people to tell me what to do; wouldn't like to be the boss. I like pleasing myself though – like my routines. I could live happily on my own I think.

Peer Approval

Jean is a great encouragement. She says I'll get over this – its just a bad patch. Dick was always on at me to pull myself together, see a doctor, do something!

Family Approval

Dad used to compliment me on my cooking. Mother never does anything but criticise and complain.

Success

I never wanted success, not for myself. I always wanted Dick to do well though. I like to do things well – like cooking or gardening. Spend a lot of time on that. I hate being criticised. (again)

Personal Appraisal

I am loyal and hard-working. Wouldn't like people to think I'm putting all this on.

PREFERENCE RANKING

1) Encouragement from Mum
   (if possible)
2) More independence
3) Jean's encouragement

1) Criticism
2) Too much responsibility
3) Feeling that I'm a total failure.

– 6 –

SELF-CONTROL POTENTIAL

┌——— Control ———┐

Asset	Overt	Covert
Lost over a stone in weight last year.	Kept a card in my bag saying what I could and couldn't eat.	Kept 'thinking thin' when I was tempted. Praised myself whenever I was tempted and resisted.

SOCIAL RELATIONSHIPS

Significant Other	Relationship	Role
Mr. Jameson	Church Minister	Support & encouragement
Jean Davidson	Friend	Encouragement
Dr. Sommers	General Practitioner	Support (? too much)
? Mother		Encouragement.

THERAPEUTIC EXPECTATIONS

I want you to help me get over this. Just tell me what to do and I'll do it. I've been on just about every drug you can name and its doing me no good. You're my last hope.

* Discourage passive role.

– 7 –

ASSESSMENT	TARGET	METHOD
	Assertiveness	Rathus Ass. Inventory (given 19/11/80)
	Social skills (v. & non v) in role-play	Direct observation in clinic.
	anxiety	Fear survey schedule (given 19/11/80)
MODIFICATION	Coping with criticism	Assertion training
	Coping with crowds	Stress inoculation training in clinic
	decrease anxiety	exposure <u>in vivo</u>

SUMMARY   Mrs. Smith complains of anxiety and panic attacks when in crowds (e.g. shops, at work). However she also experiences this problem when under stress in smaller social settings (e.g. handling clients, being criticised or having heavy demands made on her). She gets flustered, feels her legs weaken and her heart pounding. Usually she takes flight – hiding in toilet or rushing home. As soon as she has escaped she feels better : but later suffers recriminations. This problem has been growing steadily for a number of years (? date of promotion to private secretary). She used to go out socially until her father died (brief depressive episode). Her husband used to 'force her' to go out with him only making matters worse.

   She has a number of 'supports' – her friend (J.D.) is realistic and gives good advice. She tends to be passive and wants me to cure her. Much of her anxiety appears to be fuelled by 'negative thinking.'   * Discuss medication with G.P.
          Hierarchy next session
       ? Social skills group at Day Hospital
       Will Mother make good co-therapist or Jean Davidson

APPENDIX 2: GENERAL ASSESSMENT SYSTEMS

The Assessment of Anxiety or Fear

A number of Fear Survey Schedules (FSS) have been developed to assess the patient's typical reaction to a broad range of 'fearful' situations. The patient is asked to rate his fear of a number of different experiences or situations, using either a five-point or seven-point rating scale. The scale assesses items such as 'dogs, dead bodies, heart palpitations' from 'no fear' through to 'terror' or 'complete avoidance'. The patient may complete this scale as a homework assignment.

Reference: Wolpe, J. and Lang, P.J. 'A fear survey schedule for use in behaviour therapy', *Behaviour Research and Therapy*, vol. 2 (1964), pp. 27-30.

The Assessment of Assertive Behaviour

A number of rating scales measure assertive behaviour. The patient is asked to indicate how characteristic a number of statements are of his behaviour, e.g. 'I often have a hard time saying no', or 'When I am given a compliment I sometimes just don't know what to say'. This scale is completed independently by the patient.

Reference: Rathus, S.A. 'A 30 item schedule for assessing assertive behaviour', *Behaviour Therapy*, vol. 4 (1973), pp. 398-406.

The Assessment of Social Anxiety

Two scales have been developed to assess social anxiety. The Social Avoidance and Distress (SAD) Scale measures the experience of distress, discomfort and anxiety in social situations. The Fear of Negative Evaluation (FNE) Scale assesses the extent to which the patient is apprehensive about criticism or disapproval from others in social situations.

Reference: Watson, D. and Friend, R. 'Measurement of social-evaluative anxiety', *Journal of Consulting and Clinical Psychology*, vol. 32 (1969), pp. 448-57.

The Assessment of Chronic Psychiatric Patients

A number of rating scales have been developed to provide a broad overview of the hospitalised patient. One of the best known is the Nurses Observation Scale for Inpatients (NOSIE). Staff rate the patient over a period of three days, giving scores on items such as social competence, social interest, neatness, irritability, manifest psychosis and retardation.

Reference: Honigfeld, G., Gillis, R.O. and Klett, C.J. 'NOSIE – 30: a treatment sensitive ward behaviour scale', *Psychological Reports*, vol. 19 (1966), pp. 180–2.

The Mentally Handicapped

An adaptive behaviour scale (ABS) is available for children and adults. This assesses a broad range of appropriate and inappropriate behaviour. In the first part of the scale adaptive behaviours – such as dressing, money handling, language and social skills – are assessed. In part two, maladaptive behaviours – such as violence, withdrawal and self-injury – are assessed. The scale has over 400 individual items and can take some time to complete. However, the overview provided is truly comprehensive.

Reference: AAMD 'Adaptive Behaviour Scale' (Washington, DC, American Association on Mental Deficiency, 1974).

The Assessment of Everyday Living Skills

The Everyday Living Skills Inventory (ELSI) was developed to assess performance across a range of 86 everyday behaviours. Using a six-point rating scale the patient is assessed on items such as: dressing and walking, at the basic level; social interaction and play, at the intermediate level; and shopping and using public services, on the highest level. The scores are translated on to visual profiles (see Figure A2.1) which illustrate the patient's areas of ability and disability. The scale has been used with mentally handicapped children and adults, some chronic psychiatric patients and the elderly.

Reference: Barker, P., Tosh, M. and Spooner, B., 'The everyday living skills inventory: a field trial of a global nursing assessment package. Manuscript submitted for publication. (Note: Copies of ELSI are available from the author.)

Figure A2.1: ELSI — A Global Assessment

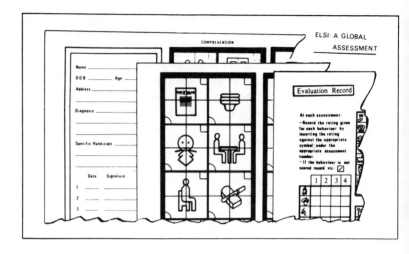

APPENDIX 3: ETHICAL GUIDELINES

The following guidelines are suggested for use by nurses who are engaged in behaviour therapy. The guidelines are appropriate for the nurse who is involved in the direction and planning of a programme and also for the nurse conducting the treatment. These guidelines are not absolute, nor are they all-encompassing. Care or treatment may involve considerations which are not covered by the points which follow.

The main aim of the ethical guidelines is to provide a simple structure which should *help* exclude the danger of any infringement of the legal and human rights of the patient.

(1) Assessment. The first stage of therapy involves the identification of the patient's problem. Every attempt should be made to:

(a) Ensure that a *comprehensive* assessment is carried out as a matter of routine. The patient's problem should be studied within the perspective of his overall functioning.
(b) Assess each patient *individually* and *objectively*, by comparison with people of his own age, and from similar social and cultural backgrounds, where appropriate.
(c) Assess the role of the patient's physical and social *environment* in terms of any contribution it may make to the problem under review.
(d) Assess each problem in the light of the patient's future, as well as immediate circumstances.

(2) Aims of Treatment. The second stage of therapy involves the design of the treatment programme and the setting of immediate *objectives* which will lead to the final *aim* of the programme. At this stage every attempt should be made to:

(a) Ensure that any aims or objectives are based upon a close evaluation of the assessment information.
(b) Ensure that all aims and objectives are in the best interests of the patient.
(c) Ensure that stages in the development of the programme lead, logically, to the final aim of treatment.

263

(d) Ensure that the final aim — and objectives — are defined clearly and recorded for discussion, *before* any decision to begin treatment is taken.

(3) Consent. The patient should be given the chance to give, or withold, his consent to the treatment. Where he cannot exercise consent appropriately, someone should represent the patient. In general, this role would be undertaken by the medical officer responsible for the patient's overall care. In other cases it may be the patient's next of kin. Every attempt should be made to:

(a) Ensure that the patient, or his representative, is aware of the *details* of the programme before his consent is requested. Ideally, aims and objectives should be prepared in some appropriate format, for discussion purposes.
(b) Ensure that consent is given freely, excluding any suggestion of coercion, no matter how subtle.
(c) Offer a choice of treatment strategies, or aims of treatment, wherever appropriate.
(d) Allow the patient to discontinue the programme without suffering any costs which he, or his representative, had not been informed of initially.
(e) Make changes in the programme *only* after receiving the approval of the patient or his representative.

(4) Treatment Methods. In selecting the techniques which will be used to achieve the aims of treatment, attempt to ensure that:

(a) The methods selected are of specific relevance to the patient's problem.
(b) The treatment methods have a degree of 'respectability'. Wherever possible, use techniques which have been shown to be successful in resolving the kind of problem presented.
(c) Any costs to the patient, either financial, physical or emotional, are outweighed by the benefits likely to be gained.
(d) Any controversial technique likely to be used has been approved by the patient's responsible medical officer and the appropriate senior nursing representative.

(5) Evaluation. The treatment programme should be monitored closely from the outset. Every attempt should be made to:

(a) Ensure that a reliable and valid assessment of the patient's problems is undertaken before, and during, the treatment.
(b) Ensure that all assessment information is analysed carefully in order to correct, or stop, an ineffective or inappropriate programme, at the earliest opportunity.
(c) Ensure that evaluation information is available at any time for study by the patient or his representative.

(6) The Change-agent.   The success of the programme is influenced greatly by the expertise and motivation of the nurse involved. Every attempt should be made to:

(a) Ensure that the nurse has had experience and training in the methods involved in the programme and in relation to the presenting problem, wherever possible.
(b) Ensure that the nurse is aware of the reporting procedure and of her responsibility for abiding by such a rule.
(c) Ensure that inexperienced nurses have an adequate back-up from specialist staff, from any profession, and the support of an appropriate organisational structure.
(d) Ensure that the patient is offered specialist help, where this is available, or the nature of the problem demands this.

APPENDIX 4: PROGRAMME ASSESSMENT, PLANNING AND EVALUATION RECORD (PAPER)

Name . . . .
Resident in . . . .
Supervisor . . . .

Sign and date
each stage as
it is completed.

	Date	Signature
1. Receipt of referral.	____	_____
2. Open/re-open case file.	____	_____
3. Define referred problem (s).	____	_____
4. Complete cost-benefit analysis.	____	_____
5. Discuss cost-benefit analysis with significant others — reach decision.	____	_____
6. Conduct problem-oriented interview.	____	_____
7. Conduct preliminary observation of patient.	____	_____
8. Conduct global assessment, where appropriate.	____	_____
9. Prepare preliminary report on 1–8.	____	_____
10. Discuss report with significant others.	____	_____
11. Set treatment goals or discharge case.	____	_____
12. Prepare baseline measure/set in operation.	____	_____
13. Evaluate baseline: e.g. graph.	____	_____
14. Design treatment programme: summarise stages and procedures briefly.	____	_____
15. Discuss programme with significant others.	____	_____
16. Assess ethical implications: adjust programme accordingly.	____	_____
17. Discuss organisation of programme with significant others: adjust accordingly.	____	_____
18. Prepare monitoring format.	____	_____
19. Fulfil training needs where appropriate.	____	_____
20. Gain consent to begin treatment programme.	____	_____
21. Commence treatment programme.	____	_____
22. Evaluate Treatment records.	____	_____
23. Discuss progress or alteration of programme with significant others.	____	_____
24. Revise programme if target not reached.	____	_____
	____	_____
	____	_____
	____	_____
	____	_____
	____	_____
	____	_____
25. Discontinue programme: failure.	____	_____
26. Begin phase-out of programme: success.	____	_____
27. Complete phase-out of programme.	____	_____
28. Notify all staff of end of programme.	____	_____
29. Thank all for assistance and co-operation.	____	_____
30. Return any equipment borrowed.	____	_____
31. Complete analysis of treatment records.	____	_____
32. Prepare the final report.	____	_____
33. Submit report to all significant staff.	____	_____
34. Return notes to case file.	____	_____
35. Follow up case at appropriate date.	____	_____

APPENDIX 5: RELAXATION TRAINING

General Instructions

The following instructions can be given by the nurse initially, and then transferred to an audio-tape for private use by the patient. The instructions represent only a *guide* to the major steps in training. In the first session it may be helpful for the nurse to practise the steps along with the patient, pacing the instructions to suit him and pointing out the feelings which *she* is experiencing – e.g. 'feel how the tension runs right up your forearm' or 'feel how heavy your arms have become'. The patient should be warned that he may not feel relaxed right away and may feel a little uncomfortable after the first session.

Situation

The patient is told to practise the exercises in the same situation each time, at first. This should be in a warm room, softly lit, without too many distractions. Absolute quietness is artificial and unnecessary. The patient can adopt either a lying or sitting position, whichever he prefers. If lying, he should lie on a rug rather than a bed, with a pillow under his head. If sitting, an armchair – which supports arms and head and allows the feet to rest comfortably on the floor – should be used. (The instructions below use an armchair.)

Preparation

Before beginning the nurse should check that the patient does not have any physical problem which might interfere with the training (e.g. muscle injury). This region would be isolated from the instructions. The nurse tells the patient what she wants him to do and how long the session will last. Finally she advises him against straining too hard in the tension parts of the exercises; this is particularly indicated in respect of the neck exercises.

Steps in Training

(1)   Take a deep breath through your nose, and hold it. (Pause 10 seconds) Now breathe out slowly. Carry on breathing gently . . . in . . . (following the patient's rhythm) . . . and out.

(2)   Raise your arms in front of you. Continue breathing normally. Make a tight fist with each hand. Study the feeling of tension . . . in your hands . . . running up your wrist and forearm. Study that feeling of tension until I count to three . . . and then let your hands drop back down on to the chair. One . . . two . . . three.

(3)   Rest your arm on the arm of the chair. Keep the heel of your hand resting on the arm and stretch your fingers as wide as they will go. Continue stretching . . . feel your fingers and thumbs pulling apart. Stop stretching and let your hands settle back on the arm.

(4)   Raise both arms in front of you and flap your hands. Shake them loose. Let the shaking run right up your forearm . . . let your elbows go loose too. And let them settle back on the arm.

(5)   Pull your shoulders down towards your feet. Keep your arms relaxed. Just study the feeling as you pull your shoulders down. Feel the tightness in your shoulders . . . and stop.

(6)   Hunch your shoulders up into your neck. Pull them up as far as they will go. Keep both arms relaxed. And drop them again.

(7)   Arch your shoulders backwards . . . pulling the shoulder blades together. Feel the tightness in your shoulder blades and across your chest. And stop . . . let your shoulders drop again.

(8)   Let your head roll to the left side. Let it fall away as far as it will go. Feel the tightness running up the right side of your neck. And let your head come back into its natural position.

(9)   Let your head roll to the right side. Let it fall away as far as it will go. Feel the tightness running up the left side of your neck. And let your head come back into its natural position.

(10)   Push your head back into the chair. Study the feeling of tension in your throat and neck. And . . . relax.

(11)   Let your head fall on to your chest. Let it hang further . . . and further down. Feel the tension running up the back of your neck. And relax . . . letting your head come back to its normal position.

(12)   Keeping your lips together, pull your jaw downwards . . . separating your teeth. Study the feeling of tension in your lower jaw and across your face. And gently . . . relax.

(13)   Press your lips together . . . study the feeling which runs from your lips back through your cheeks. And relax. Study the feeling of

warmth and looseness in . . . and around your lips and mouth.

(14) Push your tongue up into the roof of your mouth. Hold it there and study the tension running back down your tongue into your throat. And . . . relax . . . letting your tongue settle on to the floor of your mouth.

(15) Press your tongue against the back of your teeth. Again feel the tension inside your tongue and in your throat. And relax.

(16) Close your eyes tightly. Screw them up. Feel the tightness circling around them. And relax.

(17) Open your eyes as wide as they will go . . . wrinkling your forehead at the same time. Pull your eyebrows up . . . up as high as they will go. And relax. Let your eyelids settle and your forehead slacken.

(18) Tighten the whole of the top of your body . . . shoulders, arms, neck, face. And relax.

(19) Take a deep breath. And hold it. And relax . . . letting the whole of your upper body relax.

(20) Tense your stomach muscles. Feel that tension running right up through your chest into your throat. And relax.

(21) Tighten your buttocks, pressing your back against the chair. Study the feelings around your buttocks, thighs and lower back. And relax.

(22) Push both feet firmly against the floor. Feel the tension in your knees and thighs. Feel the tightness running from your thighs into your hips. And relax.

(23) Raise your toes up towards your face. Feel the tension running up your shins from your ankles. And relax.

(24) Press both knees together and tense your whole lower body: feet, legs, hips. Study that tension. And relax. Let yourself go loose.

(25) That now completes the training. I want you now to take a deep breath . . . and hold it . . . and breathe out. Good. Now I want you to check over your whole body . . . seeking out any little areas of tension. Start from your hands where they are resting on the arms of the chair . . . up your forearms to your elbows. Check out your upper arms and shoulders . . . through your shoulders to your back and up your neck into your head and face. Check down over the front of your chest and your stomach . . . down into your hips. Loosen your buttocks and let yourself sink more into the seat. Run a check down your thighs, your knees and down towards your feet and toes. Wiggle your toes a bit, just to loosen them that bit more. I want you now to sit for about a minute, just let yourself *sit back*: don't try to relax. When I count three I want you to open your eyes feeling nice . . . and comfortable . . . and relaxed. One . . . two . . . three.

GLOSSARY

ABAB design. An experimental design used to evaluate the effects of treatment on the target behaviour. In phase A the behaviour is assessed under baseline conditions. In phase B the treatment is introduced. In the second A phase the baseline is reintroduced and in the second B phase the treatment is reintroduced.

Antecedent. The stimulus event which precedes the behaviour.

Assertiveness. Standing up for one's rights: the proper expression of any emotion, other than anxiety, towards another person. Often called *assertion.*

Aversive event. Anything which *suppresses* the behaviour which it follows (punishment) or *increases* the behaviour which is performed to terminate it (negative reinforcement).

Avoidance. Acting in a way which postpones or prevents the occurrence of an aversive event.

Back-up reinforcer. Any object or activity which can be obtained in exchange for tokens earned within a token economy system.

Backward chaining. A technique for developing a sequence of behaviours by teaching the last part of the chain first. The next to last behaviour in the chain is taught second and so on back through the chain, until the person can complete the whole sequence.

Baseline. The initial assessment period of a behavioural programme in which the patient's behaviour is studied under natural or non-treatment conditions.

Behaviour rehearsal. Imaginal or actual practice of the target behaviour in preparation for performing this in the natural environment.

Classical conditioning. A type of associative learning in which a neutral stimulus is paired with an unconditioned stimulus which elicits a reflex behaviour automatically. After repeated pairing of the neutral and unconditioned stimuli, the neutral stimulus acquires the power to elicit the reflex behaviour also.

Conditioned reinforcer. A secondary reinforcer; any object or activity which acquires reinforcing properties through learning, i.e. as a result of pairing with an existing reinforcer.

Conditioned response. A reflex behaviour which is elicited by a conditioned stimulus, where the unconditioned stimulus is absent.

Conditioned stimulus. A previously neutral stimulus which has acquired the power to elicit a conditioned response by repeated association with an unconditioned stimulus.

Consequence. The stimulus event which follows the behaviour.

Contingency. The relationship between a behaviour and its outcome.

Contingency contract. A formal agreement between people who wish someone's behaviour to change (e.g. parents, spouse, nurses) and the person whose behaviour is to change (e.g. children, spouse, patient). The contract specifies the consequences which will follow the performance of specified desired or undesired behaviours, by each party.

Continuous reinforcement. A reinforcement schedule in which every consecutive response is reinforced.

Cost-benefit analysis. An evaluation of the pros and cons of any treatment programme: in particular, weighing up the costs likely to be involved (effort, time, etc.) and the benefits likely to be gained.

270

Co-therapist. A supporting therapist used where more than one patient is involved, e.g. marital therapy, group therapy.

Covert behaviour. Private events – such as thinking, fantasies, imagination – which are observable only by the person experiencing them.

Cue. The discriminative stimulus which signals that reinforcement will follow a certain response.

Delayed reinforcement. A technique for fading reinforcement by gradual extension of the time between the performance of the behaviour and the delivery of reinforcement.

Deprivation. The state in which the individual is denied access to reinforcement.

Differential reinforcement of other behaviours (DRO). A technique for reducing maladaptive behaviour in which any behaviour *except* the target maladaptive behaviour is reinforced.

Discrimination. Behaving differently in response to different cues.

Discrimination training. Teaching a person to recognise (discriminate) when it is appropriate or inappropriate to perform certain behaviours.

Duration record. A measure of how long a person spends engaged in a behaviour.

Elicit. To bring about a behaviour automatically: e.g. a reflex behaviour, such as blinking in bright light.

Emit. To behave voluntarily (e.g. operant behaviour).

Escape training. A negative reinforcement technique in which the patient performs the target behaviour in order to remove or stop an aversive event.

Experimental design. The plan of the treatment programme which allows evaluation of specific treatment methods. The commonest designs are reversals (ABAB) and multiple baseline design.

Extinction. A technique for reducing behaviour, in which the reinforcer is *not given* for a previously reinforced behaviour.

Fading. The gradual removal of prompts which are used to signal or assist the performance of a behaviour. It is used often to refer to the 'thinning out' of reinforcement on a reinforcement schedule.

Fixed-interval. A reinforcement schedule in which the first behaviour to occur after a specified time has elapsed, is reinforced.

Fixed-ratio. A reinforcement schedule in which reinforcement is given only after a specified number of behaviours have been performed.

Flooding. A technique for reducing avoidance behaviour in which the patient is required to remain in the feared situation for long periods of time. Often called *prolonged exposure.*

Frequency count. A measure of how often a behaviour is shown within a specific period of time.

Fuzzy. A description of the patient's behaviour which does not specify what he says or does, but is a projection of the observer's view of the behaviour.

Generalisation. Behaving in the same way in situations which are similar to those under which the behaviour was first learned.

High-probability behaviour (HPB). A behaviour which is performed regularly when the person is free to choose one of several behavioural options.

Hierarchy. An arrangement, or list, of items, events or situations, in order of avoidance or fearfulness. Items at the bottom of the hierarchy are avoided or feared only a little; those at the top are avoided or feared greatly. Used in the treatment plan for avoidance behaviour.

Incompatible behaviour. One behaviour which cannot occur at the same time as another behaviour.

Intermittent reinforcement. A reinforcement schedule in which only some occurrences of the behaviour are reinforced. (See Fixed interval and ratio.)

Latency recording. A measure of how long a person takes to perform a given behaviour, from the first appearance of the cue for the action to take place.

Low-probability behaviour (LPB). A behaviour which is performed rarely, when the person is free to choose from one of several behavioural options.

Mediational processes. The hypothetical 'internal events' – e.g. thought, attention, memory – which link the performance of a behaviour with the events in the environment which originally led to its occurrence.

Medical model. The view that maladaptive behaviour is caused by underlying processes. The problem behaviour is seen as a symptom of some psychological 'disease'.

Modelling. A technique where one person (the model) demonstrates the target behaviour in order to allow imitation to take place.

Multiple baseline design. An experimental design in which the treatment is applied to different behaviours, or across different situations, over a period of time.

Negative reinforcement. A means of strengthening behaviour by removal of an aversive event contingent upon the performance of the target behaviour.

Observational learning. Learning by observing someone else (the model) and observing the outcome. Often called *vicarious learning.*

Operant behaviour. Behaviour which is controlled by its consequences: voluntary behaviour.

Operant conditioning. A type of associative learning in which the behaviour is influenced by alteration of the consequences which it produces.

Overcorrection. A technique for reducing behaviour in which the person must correct the consequences of his undesirable behaviour and then must practise repeating the more desirable version of the behaviour.

Overt behaviour. Behaviour which is publicly observable.

Positive reinforcement. Any consequence of a behaviour which increases the future possibility of that behaviour.

Primary reinforcer. Any event which does not depend upon learning for its reinforcing properties: e.g. food, drink, warmth, sex.

Prompt. A cue; any event (instruction, gesture, etc.) which helps initiate a behaviour.

Punishment. Any consequence which reduces the future probability of a behaviour. This usually involves the presentation of some aversive event, or removal of positive reinforcement, for a time or permanently.

Reinforcer sampling. A technique for extending a person's range of positive reinforcers (reinforcer 'menu'). The person is allowed access to the reinforcer for only a short time or is allowed to consume only a small part of it.

Reliability check. A procedure for evaluating the accuracy of an assessment measure by comparing the scores of independent observers.

Respondent behaviour. Reflex behaviour; that which is elicited by an antecedent stimulus (e.g. actions of glands or smooth muscles).

Response cost. Removal of positive reinforcement permanently, as a consequence of a behaviour; similar to fining.

Satiation. Giving positive reinforcement to excess, resulting in an aversive event.

Secondary reinforcer. Anything which acquires its reinforcing properties through association with existing reinforcers.

Self-control. Any behaviour which a person performs to increase or decrease other patterns of his own behaviour.

Self-instruction. A technique in which a person prompts himself through a specific chain of behaviours, usually done covertly.

Shaping. Building a pattern of behaviour by reinforcing successive approximations of the final target.

Socratic irony. A technique used in cognitive therapy where the therapist questions the patient as though she does not understand the patient's view of his problem. This leads him to affirm something which reveals the absurdity of his values or beliefs.

Systematic desensitisation. A technique for overcoming avoidance behaviour in which the patient's anxious response is extinguished by gradual exposure to the feared situation by use of a hierarchy. This exposure is done initially in imagination and then *in vivo* (real life).

Target behaviour. The behaviour which is to be changed in the treatment programme.

Thought-stopping. A technique which helps the patient control aversive thoughts, by saying 'Stop' subvocally to himself.

Time-out from reinforcement. The removal of reinforcement for a specified period of time in order to reduce the future probability of a behaviour.

Token economy. A reinforcement system in which conditioned reinforcers (tokens) are earned for a range of behaviours and exchanged for back-up reinforcers.

Vicarious reinforcement. The hypothetical process whereby one individual's behaviour is influenced by observing another person receiving reinforcement.

INDEX